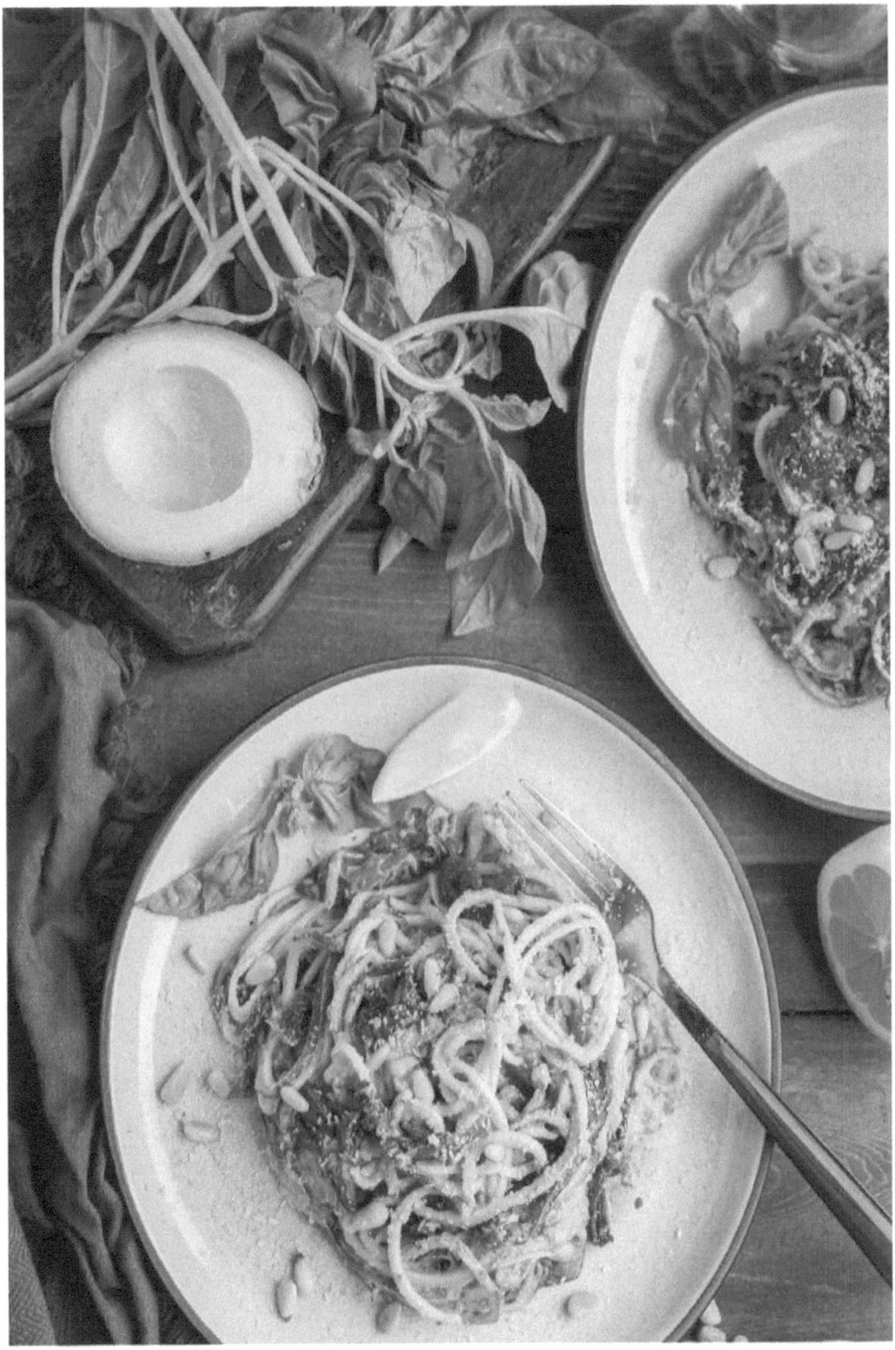

AF439902

CONTENTS

Baked Tortilla Chips
Pesto Essential Goat Cheese Spread
Garlic-Herb Popcorn
Salt and Pepper Kale Chips
Tabbouleh
Slow Cooker Apple Sauce
Chocolate-Almond Dip with Strawberries

VEGETARIAN DINNER

Vegetarian Chili
Grilled Mini Veggie Pizzas
Mushroom Barley Risotto
Chinese Cashew Chicken
Rice Noodles with Ginger Salmon
Creole Red Beans and Rice
Curried Chickpeas with Spinach and Brown Rice
Vietnamese Tofu Lettuce Wraps
Vegetable Fried Rice

MEAT & SEAFOOD

Spice-Rubbed Salmon with Citrus Salsa and Steamed Asparagus
Shrimp Succotash
Mighty Mushroom and Tilapia Seafood Dinner
Honey-Tamari Salmon with Rice and Snow Peas
Steamed Mussels in Tomato-Fennel Broth
Chicken Pasta Puttanesca
Tandoori Chicken Kabobs
Pork and Bok Choy Stir-Fry
Chicken and Broccoli Tetrazzini

DESSERTS

Banana Cookie with Choko Chips
Lemon-Lime Granita
Broiled Grapefruit with Honeyed Yogurt
Apple Crumble
Apple-Raisin Rice Pudding
Yogurt Cheesecake Bars with Berry Topping
Quick Vanilla Pudding

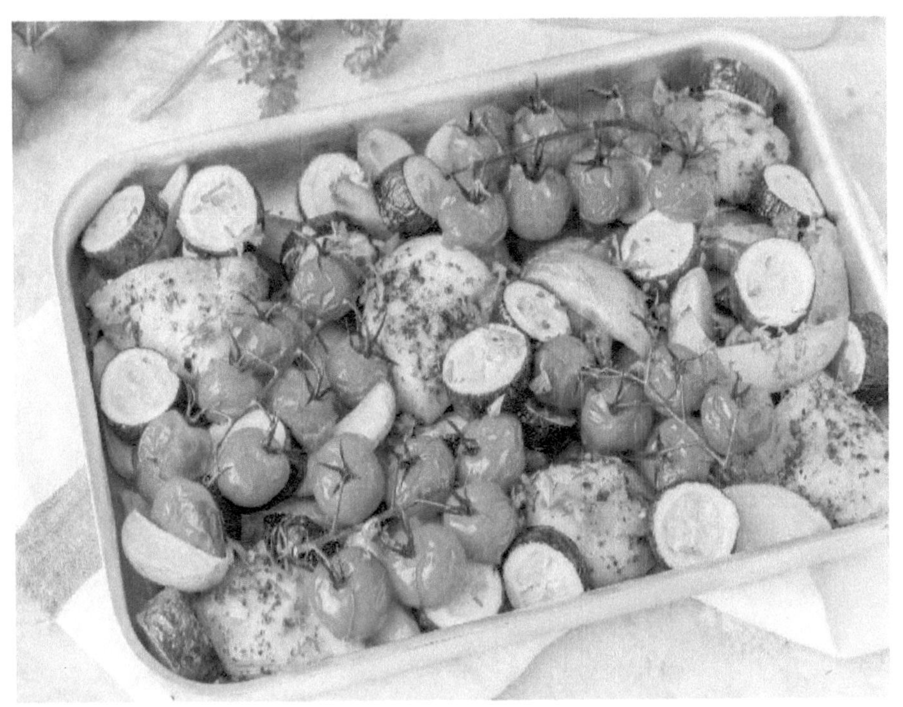

INTRODUCTION

For most, food is pleasure. We indulge in it as much as we can and as much as we need. But have you ever stopped to consider whether that greasy hamburger is worth wearing around your stomach? Have you ever thought about how many calories a friend's chocolate birthday cake would give you? If yes, then you might just be considering making a change in your diet to help you become healthier.

Clean eating has becoming increasingly popular. After years of fueling ourselves with junk food, processed fillers, and refined sugars, our society has fallen to obesity, cancer, heart disease, depression, anxiety, and so many other ailments that decrease our overall life expectancy and quality of life. In a sense, we are killing ourselves with the foods we choose on a daily basis. And it must stop.

Note that clean eating brings "health" beyond anything else. It doesn't ask you to reduce your calories; it doesn't ask you to reduce your overall carbohydrate content. It doesn't even ask you to stop eating dessert, although refined sugars are eliminated, replaced only with nature's most delightful natural sugars. It stresses principles that are rooted in nutritional science, that bring overall enhanced vitamins and minerals to your daily life.

Clean eating is a lifestyle which many experts believe to be one of the main reasons people stay in top shape. From this book you'll learn about clean eating, including its benefits, how to start eating clean, clean eating recipes, and much more. You will be surprised at how much the clean eating diet can benefit you.

What is Eating Clean?

The "clean eating" diet plan isn't really a diet at all. Instead, it is an alteration in the way you think about your food. Instead of eliminating one type of food from your diet—like carbohydrates or fats—you work to better understand the route your food took from its origin to its final place in your body, helping you to both lose weight and create lasting energy.

Essentially, clean eating allows you to eat whole foods, unprocessed foods, and foods that have not been altered on their way to your refrigerator or freezer. Through the clean eating mindset, you learn to refuse refined and processed foods. However, because our current society handles food on such a complex level these days, eating clean can be an incredibly challenging nutritional approach.

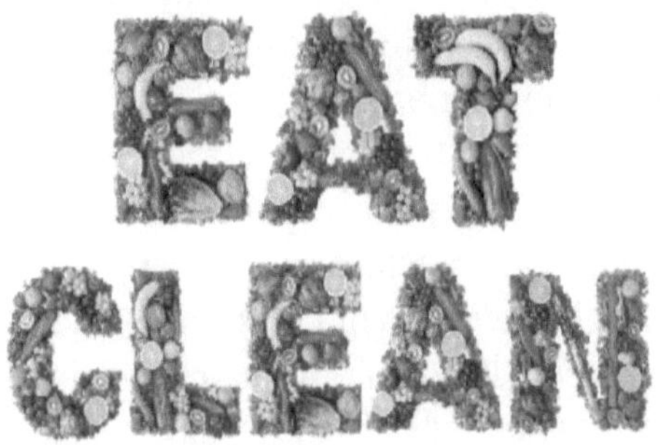

Whole foods grow in the garden, roam freely on farms, or swim in the sea. Think about the food chain you learned about during your science classes. Single-celled animals, plants, and plankton are at the bottom. Small fish and other tiny animals eat the single-celled animals, and bigger animals eat the small fish and other tiny animals, and so on up the chain. People (and sharks) are at the top, so everything eaten by the creatures lower on the chain becomes part of the creatures at the top.

To understand all the health benefits of eating clean, you need to consider another food chain: the processed food chain. A plain apple, a handful of chickpeas, or an organic egg are at the bottom. As you move further up the chain, manufacturers manipulate the food until it becomes more artificial ingredients than real food. The foods at the top of this chain include traditional snack foods, fast food, and foods packed with additives, preservatives, and artificial flavors.

Manufacturers end up stripping processed foods of many of their nutrients either to make them easier to combine with other ingredients or to change their characteristics. In contrast, whole foods come to you just as nature intended—bursting with flavor, color, texture, and nutrients.

The foods that are part of the eating clean plan are at the bottom of the processed food chain. They don't have labels, they don't carry preparation instructions, and they certainly don't have ingredient lists. These are the foods to buy each time you go to the supermarket

What Does "Processed" Food Look Like?

In order to understand how to initiate the clean eating diet plan, it is essential to know your enemy. Stay away from processed foods:

1. Processed foods have additions of all kinds. They have added fat, salt, sugar, or preservatives. Note that these preservatives work to keep the food "fresher" for longer. However, you do not want to put those additives in your body.
2. Processed foods have been altered from their traditional state. Look, for example, at whole grains without their initial germ or bran. This created refined bread, which is quite popular on the market, even though it is relatively void of nutrients.
3. Processed foods have lab-manufactured ingredients. Generally, you'll find these ingredients with many syllables. These ingredients are most often difficult to pronounce.

Processed foods are everywhere—from a Pop Tart to a more "healthful" packet of oatmeal. They are generally void of nutrients, and they are doing nothing for your waistline.

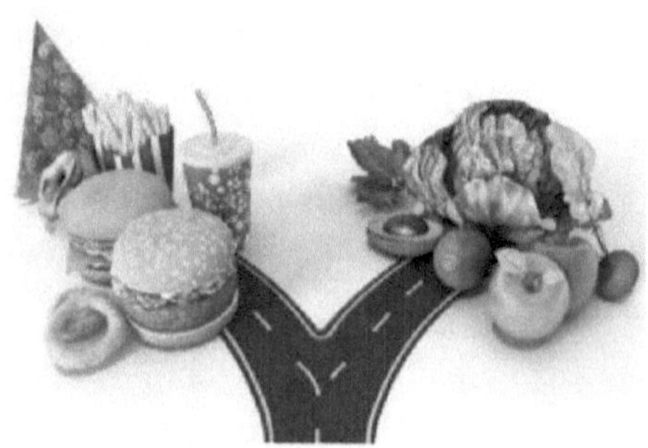

Immense Benefits of Eating Clean

Choosing to eat clean has incredible benefits, many of which are not rooted in the number on the scale. Generally speaking, slimming down in and of itself has many overarching benefits, bringing you decreased risks of developing cancers, heart diseases, depression, and anxiety. However, once many people begin clean eating, they find themselves fueled with nourishment that brings extensive benefits beyond the realms of weight loss.

1. Better ability to sleep and decreased risk of insomnia

Studies have shown the immense overall link between wellness and better sleeping habits. Many people, all over the world, struggle with sleep disturbances. Thusly, they struggle with certain diseases, they gain weight more easily, and they live a lower quality of life.

When you begin the clean eating diet, you will be able to fall asleep faster and stay asleep longer. A recent Taiwan-based four-week study notes that people with frequent problems sleeping who ate two pieces of fruit sixty minutes prior to going to sleep had better sleep quality, fell asleep about thirty percent more quickly, and slept for thirteen percent longer than normal.

It is essential to begin eating cleanly and fuel your body with essential nutrients that work to calm your inflammation and your rushing mind. They help you "shut down," in a sense, which is essential for nightly repair.

2. Better ability to stay in a happy mood

Your mood alters everything you do, the relationships you have with your family, and how you treat others. If you're in a bad mood, the quality of life you receive back from people in your life will not be incredibly high.

If you want to bring a better overall mood to your mind and your outlook, you might want to boost your produce intake. A recent New Zealand-based study notes that when you eat more vegetables and fruits, you feel calmer, have greater boosts of energy, and feel happier.

Just one no-produce day will not produce a poor mood the next day, either. The same research states that if you generally eat produce, your better mood will follow you into the next day as well.

A study posted in the Social Indicators Research journal states that when you have approximately seven servings of fruit and vegetables per day, your mood is automatically boosted. Just eating fruit can make life better, boost your perspective, and help you create better relationships with people.

3. Better ability to exercise efficiently

When you reap the rewards of clean eating, you allow yourself to build appropriate muscles, boost your ability to do longer and longer workouts, and thus burn more calories and allow your muscles to recover more quickly.

4. Better ability to function on a neurological level

Clean eating has been linked with a boost in brain function, enhancing neuron growth and communication. A study posted by the National Institutes of Nutrition states that people who ate the Clean Eating Diet and the Mediterranean diet had less brain infarcts. Brain infarcts are bits of "dead space," or dead tissue, in the brain that can ultimately lead to thought process interruptions and serious diseases like Alzheimer's and dementia.

Further research notes that six years of clean eating brings a thirty-six percent decreased risk of having interior brain damage. It also shows a decreased risk of cognitive problems associated with aging by approximately twenty-eight percent. Another study notes an incredible forty-eight percent decreased risk of developing Alzheimer's disease. This should make every dieter's ears perk up. Clean eating is essential to promoting brain function and keeping that functionality long lasting.

5. Greater exterior glow.

Clean eating gives your skin with a healthy, vibrant glow. According to recent research from the University of Nottingham, people who had eaten more fruits and vegetables were rated more attractive than people who only had sun tans, and thus were "glowing" with false beauty.

You are precisely what you eat. You show your fruits and vegetables on the outside, and your body reacts to those fruits and vegetables on the inside, accordingly.

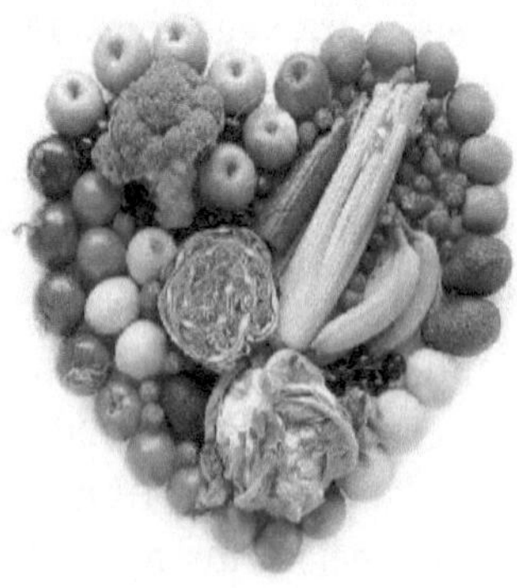

The Basics of Eating Clean

It can be hard to pull your attention away from what you're "missing out on" and focus on a delicious world of whole foods that you can eat without counting calories. But in the end, it's worth it.

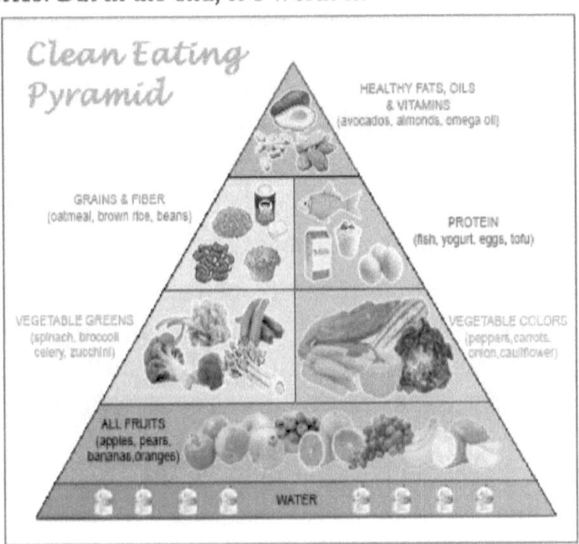

- **Stop Counting Calories**

Remember, clean eating isn't a diet. The parameters laid out in this book are flexible guidelines meant to help you find the foods you'll personally thrive on—every body is different, after all. But one thing we're pretty adamant about is that you should stop counting calories—it's unnecessary and counterproductive. As you start to cut out the junk and embrace truly nourishing foods, you'll get better in tune with your body and understand how much you need of certain foods to feel satisfied, energized, and healthy —in other words, you'll naturally self-regulate. Counting calories, on the other hand, has you focusing on a number, and often results in you feeling guilty when you don't clock in where you should at the end of the day.

- **Focus on Whole Foods**

It's time to say goodbye to highly processed convenience foods and fill your pantry and fridge with fresh, nutritious whole foods. As you begin your clean-eating journey, you'll want to stock up on a variety of fruits and vegetables, whole grains, nuts and seeds, lean proteins, and healthy fats.

These will be the pillars of your new diet and lifestyle.

- **Choose Clean Packaged Foods**

In a busy day full of work and errands, a trip to the supermarket should be one of the simpler tasks we perform. But with stores stocking more choices than ever—and with food labels making claims of everything from "more protein" to "added antioxidants"—shopping can be overwhelming. While your commitment to clean eating will ultimately make shopping easier, navigating the supermarket can feel like a challenge at first. Try to remember that the concept behind clean eating is very simple: focus on whole, unprocessed foods that contain no chemicals or other ingredients.

Also understand that, yes, sometimes it's perfectly healthy to buy food in a package. While ideally you'll strive to fill your diet with fresh fruits and vegetables and lean proteins, there are times when you may want to buy food that comes frozen or in a can or box. For example, while broccoli fresh from the farmers' market may be the healthiest pick, you'll want to have some frozen, prechopped broccoli on hand for a meal in a pinch. Tetra Paks of cooked beans, a box of whole-grain pasta, and yogurt can also be smart, minimally processed packaged choices. Of course, sometimes it's hard to determine which packaged picks are best. That's why knowing what to look for on the label can be helpful.

How to Start Eating Clean

The secret behind clean eating begins in the mind. One must have the will to start and a positive mind towards the process. Quitting some foods, especially processed foods, is not easy, it takes discipline and consistency.

1. Scrutinize Your Previous Diet

This important step will help you to cluster your foods into different categories, determining what you should throw away and what you keep. Keep those that fall under clean food and focus on them. The rest belong to the trashcan. Your health is more important than their value.

2. Make a Commitment

Transitioning from one lifestyle to another must include a commitment—in terms of time, financial resource, and shopping hours. For one to be successfully committed, there must be patience, understanding that it takes time to fully cope with the changes. Start small: instead of buying chips, go for a natural banana or an apple. Then build from there.

3. Have Strong Reasons in Mind

Leading nutritionists have stated that to change an eating habit, there must be inspiration from deep within a person. Have a motivating factor in mind when you start eating clean.

4. Shop with Reason

Processed food lasts longer because they have chemical preservatives. Buy natural foods that tell you when they need to be eaten.

5. Identify with People Who Eat Clean

It is advantageous to identify with like-minded individuals because then you will not be tempted to eat what you know is not clean.

6. Learn to Eat at Home

Food cooked outside your kitchen is cooked at high temperatures and the nutrients are lost through the heat. They are not meant to add any value to the consumer but to earn profits to the seller. When you cook your own food, you will be able to moderate it, regulate the heat, and eat without any hurry. By doing so, you will be able to choose from fresh varieties ingredients and be in a position to teach yourself to restrict your eating to clean foods.

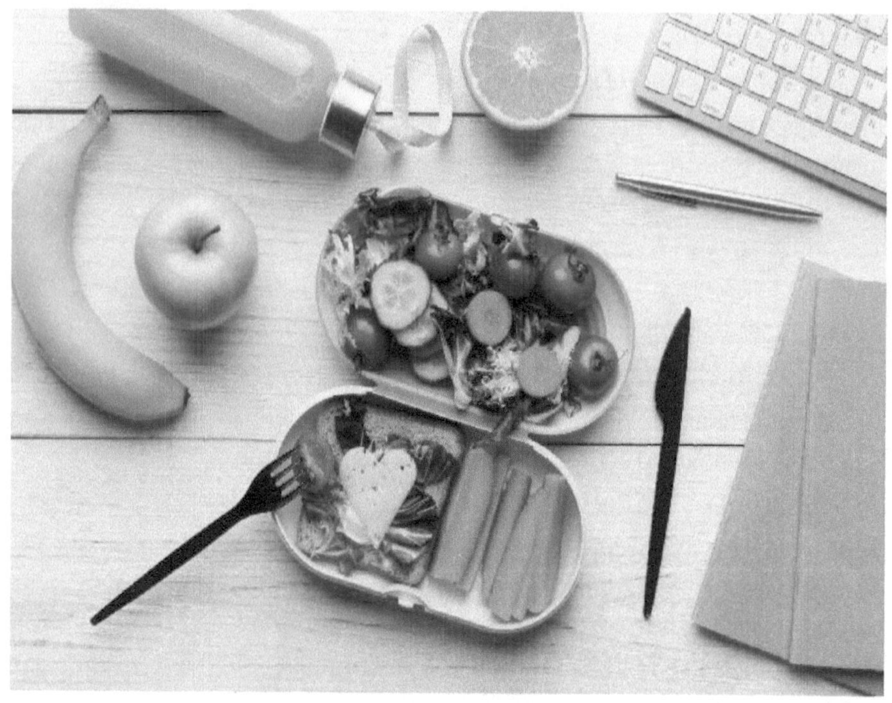

Eating Clean in a Social Setting

When at home, you choose what goes and stays in your refrigerator, which also means you will not be exposing yourself to the option of unhealthy food. When spending time at work or in a social setting, it is inevitable that you will find yourself facing a buffet table filled with fried chicken, buttered vegetables, and other food you are not used to eating anymore since you started eating clean. What should you do? Make an excuse to leave so that you can scout for a nearby grocery or health store?

Take, for example, you need to travel to attend a conference for work. Conference-goers are often provided food by the conference organizers. However, the food choices usually contain a lot of ingredients and are not really on par with the clean eating diet. While it is hard to turn down food that you know will taste good, ask yourself whether it is worth it to destroy your clean eating progress for a single serving of fried chicken. Will request for a healthier option? Or do you simply swallow your pride and eat what's served?

There is also the horror of people who think you have an eating disorder simply because you refuse to eat unhealthy food. How will you deal with these people?

While it is true that eating clean is easier to do at home, we as human beings must mingle with others.

The Office

When lunchtime comes, you could opt to visit the company cafeteria to look for something healthy to eat. However, you won't be sure of the ingredients used in preparing a seemingly healthy recipe. You can try going out, but what if the nearest health store requires you to embark on a 20-minute walk? This also means 20 minutes of your 1-hour lunchtime wasted. Well, there might be healthy snacks in the office pantry. However, chances are a huge jar of chocolate chip cookies are waiting there for you, too. What if you're hungry and you can't help but grab one? There goes your clean eating regimen.

What you should do is pack something healthy you prepared at home the morning or night before. Choose one that is quick to make and is easy to eat. Instead of bringing green salad that has a lot of ingredients, consider preparing a pre-made protein drink or have a whole-grain wrap with banana spread and mango slices in it. You can also bring grilled chicken breasts, as all you'd have to do is reheat them in the microwave.

Parties

Parties are some people's lifeblood. Refusing an invitation just because you fear there will only be unhealthy food isn't a valid reason.

If possible, check in advance what food will be served . Do not fear being branded as that diet-conscious individual who happens to be a picky eater. Just be sure to avoid going for anything that is too oily, cheesy, or melty.

If you know the host personally, ask if you can bring your own dish to share at the party. You might even be benefitting other guests by bringing a healthier alternative. Your host might also be pleased at adding something healthy to the party menu.

When it comes to alcohol, try as much as possible to refrain from gulping it down, as it only serves to provide you with unnecessary calories. Opt for one glass of wine or light beer instead.

Restaurants

An important thing to do in this social setting is to plan ahead. If you already know which restaurant your get-together will be held in, try to do some research on their menu. Most restaurants offer healthy options, so you won't have to worry about not finding one. If you can't find something perfect, settle on food that has the least number of ingredients used.

If, however, you do not find anything healthy enough for you on the menu, consider eating at home before heading out to dine with your co-workers. When you there, you can have a cup of coffee or tea. Being full, you'll be less likely to give in to the temptation of fried foods, sugary desserts, and other unhealthy food.

Should you need something in particular, don't be afraid to speak up. If you want that grilled chicken on the menu but don't want it topped with any sauce, feel free to request it.

If you want to make sure you are eating clean, relay a message to the restaurant's chefs, requesting a lower-calorie meal. Have them eliminate most of the extra added ingredients. If you want veggies, request to have them prepared minus the butter and include a salad dressing as a replacement.

The most important thing to remember when eating clean in social settings is to be as confident as possible with your decisions. You might be faced with snotty comments and nagging questions. The key is to answer in a confident tone. Once they see that you display seriousness and confidence in the lifestyle you chose, they will be less likely to bother you with their nagging in the future.

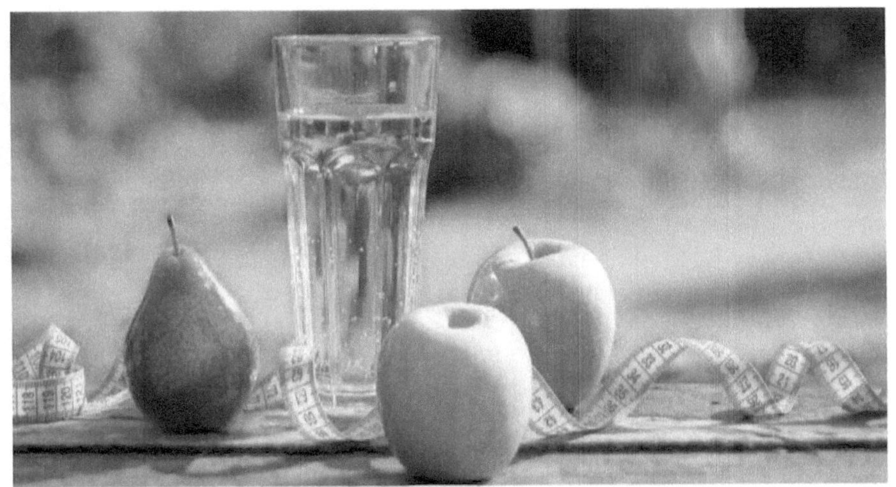

Eating Clean and the Importance of Water

When it comes to clean eating, no other liquid holds higher importance than water. Without water, the human body would not function normally since the cells will be dehydrated. Although some people might prefer fresh fruit juices to go with their clean eating diet, nothing cleanses as well as water does. This clear drink is often taken lightly because of its lack in taste. However, those who have adopted a healthy lifestyle recognize its importance to the body and make it a point to reach the recommended amount of daily water consumption.

Water is needed for all the basic functions of the human body. A good example can be seen in the very good partnership between water and the kidneys. These two are practically best friends, as water works with the kidneys in filtering out toxic waste products and bad chemicals both ingested by the body and produced by the cells. One of the biggest contributions of the kidneys is to expel urea and uric acid. To do so, there should be an adequate amount of water first so that these two can be flushed out of the body in the form of urine.

After eating your fill of the clean eating diet, it is important that your body have the capability to break down and evenly distribute the essential nutrients found in your food. Without water, both your metabolism and digestion might not be able to function well. As a result, the nutrients will not be distributed and might only get flushed out whenever you have a bowel movement.

Another benefit of making sure you get enough water can be seen in the blood. Blood is actually made up of water, and it is the water which helps in carrying the oxygen and other essential nutrients to different parts of your body, particularly the cells.

Water is also a big help to lubrication. If you suffer from dehydration, you might find it difficult to move around. Because of the lack in hydration, the joints in your body are not receiving the proper amount of lubrication they need to move freely. It also helps in lubricating the tissues inside your lungs, helping you to properly breathe.

Lastly, as human beings, we are prone to perspire whenever the weather is warm enough or whenever we perform any physical activity. If you sweat more than you drink water, you are risking dehydration. Drinking water after perspiring is a good way to refill the water levels in your body that have been lost.

So, drink water, eat clean and be healthy!

BREAKFAST

Yogurt-Berry Parfait

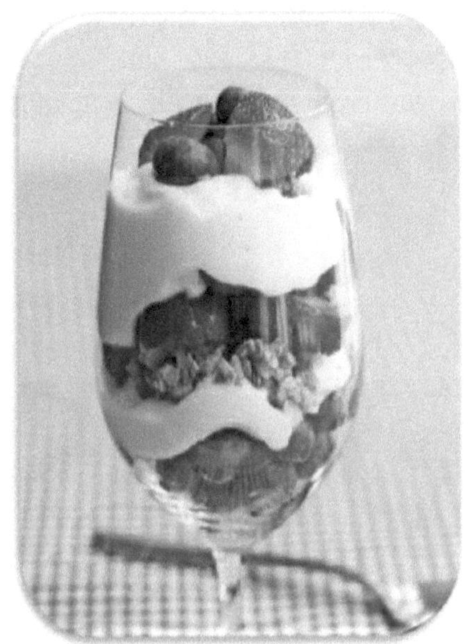

Prep time: 10 minutes
Cooking time: none
Servings: 2

Nutrients per serving:

Carbohydrates – 53.4 g
Fat – 19.9 g
Protein – 19.3 g
Calories – 235

Ingredients:

- 1 cup plain Greek yogurt
- 1 Tbsp honey
- 8 Tbsp granola with dried fruit
- ½ cup sliced strawberries
- ½ cup blueberries

Instructions:

1. In a bowl, mix the yogurt and honey.
2. Spoon ¼ cup of the yogurt mixture into each of the two serving
    bowls.
3. On top of the yogurt, sprinkle 2 Tbsp of the granola and top with ¼
    cup of the strawberries.
4. Repeat the yogurt layer and top with ¼ cup of the blueberries.
    Serve.

Pumpkin-Pecan Breakfast Cookies

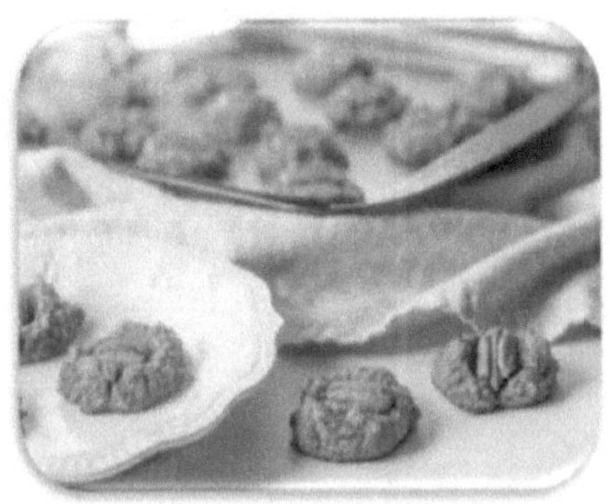

Prep time: 10 minutes
Cooking time: 20 minutes
Servings: 12

Nutrients per serving:

Carbohydrates – 10.8 g
Fat – 3.2 g
Protein – 1.8 g
Calories – 81

Ingredients:

- 1½ cups uncooked old-fashioned rolled oats
- 1 cup unsweetened canned pumpkin
- 1 cup unsweetened applesauce
- 1 cup toasted chopped pecans
- ¼ cup dried unsweetened cranberries
- 1 tsp pure vanilla extract

Instructions:

1. Preheat the oven to 350°F.
2. Line a baking sheet with parchment paper.
3. In a bowl, combine all ingredients. Let the mixture stand for 10 minutes.
4. Spoon onto the baking sheet in 12 rounds. Flatten the mounds.
5. Bake for 25 minutes.
6. Let the cookies stand for 5 minutes on the baking sheet before

removing them to cooling racks to cool completely. Serve.

Nutty Whole-Grain Waffles

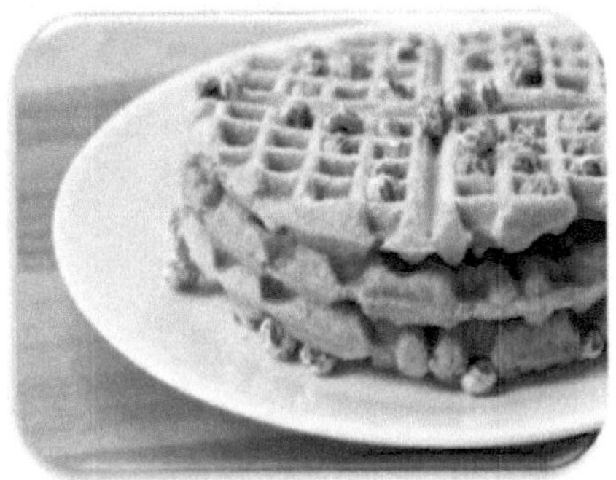

Prep time: 10 minutes
Cooking time: 5 minutes
Servings: 4

Nutrients per serving:

Carbohydrates – 67 g
Fat – 23.6 g
Protein – 7.5 g
Calories – 488

Ingredients:

- 2 eggs
- 1¾ cups unsweetened almond milk
- ¼ cup butter, plus 1 Tbsp, melted
- 2 Tbsp honey
- ½ tsp ground cinnamon
- ¼ tsp baking soda
- 1½ cups 100% whole-wheat pastry flour
- 2 tsp baking powder
- Pinch salt
- ½ cup toasted chopped pecans

Instructions:

1. Preheat a waffle iron.
2. In a bowl, mix the eggs, almond milk, ¼ cup butter, honey, cinnamon, and baking soda.

3. In another bowl, combine the flour, baking powder, salt, and pecans.
4. Add the dry ingredients to the egg mixture, whisking until combined.
5. Brush the hot waffle iron with the remaining 1 Tbsp of butter.
6. Ladle batter onto the waffle iron. Cook for 4 minutes. Repeat with the remaining batter.
7. Serve warm.

Baked Banana French Toast

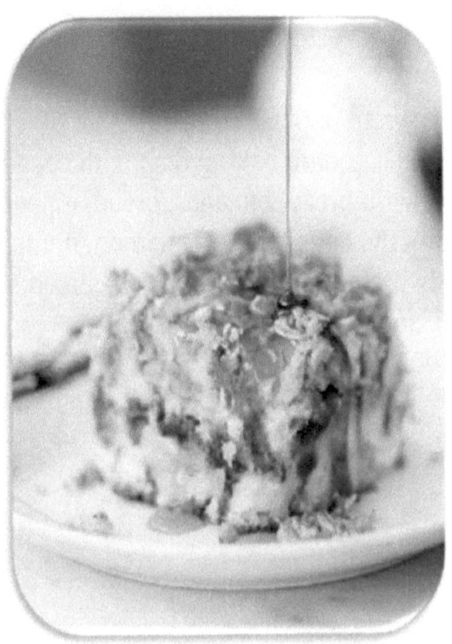

Prep time: 10 minutes
Cooking time: 45 minutes
Servings: 4

Nutrients per serving:

Carbohydrates – 53.1 g
Fat – 5.3 g
Protein – 13.8 g
Calories – 315

Ingredients:

- Coconut oil, for greasing
- 6 slices frozen sprouted-grain bread, thawed and halved
- 2 bananas, sliced
- 3 eggs
- 1½ cups milk
- ½ tsp ground cinnamon
- ¼ tsp freshly grated nutmeg
- 1 tsp pure vanilla extract
- ¼ cup coconut sugar

- Pure maple syrup, for serving

Instructions:

1. Preheat the oven to 350°F.
2. Grease an 8-inch-square baking dish with coconut oil.
3. Make a layer with bread, bananas, bread, topped with mixture.
4. In a bowl, mix the eggs, milk, cinnamon, nutmeg, vanilla, and sugar. Slowly pour the mixture over the bread slices. Press the bread to allow it to soak up the egg mixture.
5. Bake for about 50 minutes.
6. Cool slightly. Cut the casserole into servings and drizzle with the maple syrup.

Banana Nut Bread

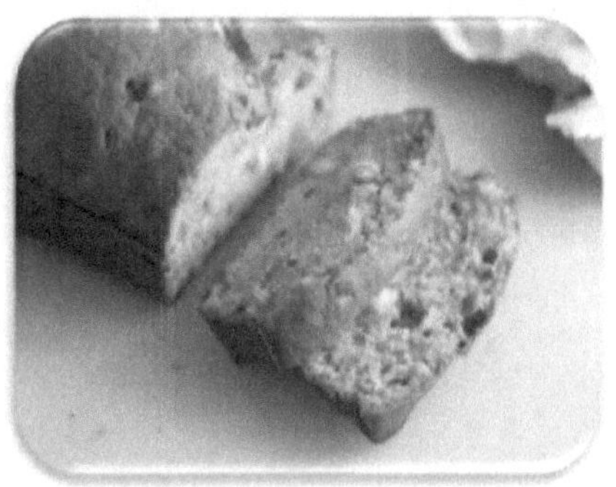

Prep time: 10 minutes
Cooking time: 45 minutes
Servings: 4

Nutrients per serving:

Carbohydrates – 17.4 g
Fat – 19.5 g
Protein – 4.9 g
Calories – 254

Ingredients:

- 1¼ cups 100% whole-wheat pastry flour
- 1 tsp baking soda
- ¼ tsp salt
- 2 eggs
- 1 tsp pure vanilla extract
- ½ cup coconut oil, plus additional for greasing pan
- ¼ cup evaporated cane juice
- 1½ cups mashed bananas (about 3 ripe)
- ½ cup toasted chopped walnuts

Instructions:

1. Preheat the oven to 350°F.
2. Coat a 9 x 5-inch loaf pan with coconut oil.
3. In a bowl, whisk the flour, baking soda, and salt.
4. In another bowl, mix the eggs, vanilla, oil, cane juice, and bananas.

5. Add the wet ingredients to the flour. Stir until combined.
6. Fold in the nuts.
7. Pour the batter into the prepared pan. Bake for about 50 minutes.
8. Remove the bread from the pan to a cooling rack and allow it to cool completely.
9. Slice and serve.

Eggs Baked in Toast Cups

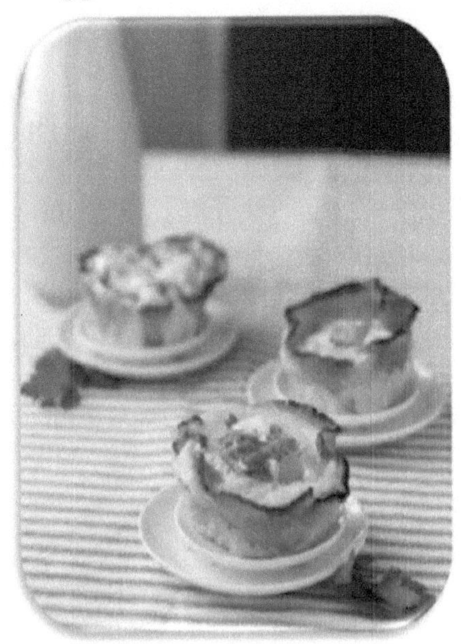

Prep time: 10 minutes
Cooking time: 20 minutes
Servings: 4

Nutrients per serving:

Carbohydrates – 16.5 g
Fat – 16 g
Protein – 13.3 g
Calories – 263

Ingredients:

- 3 Tbsp coconut oil, divided
- 4 slices frozen sprouted-grain bread, thawed
- 4 eggs
- ½ cup chopped tomato
- ½ cup shredded white Cheddar cheese
- 2 Tbsp chopped fresh basil
- ½ tsp salt
- ½ tsp freshly ground black pepper

Instructions:

1. Preheat the oven to 375°F.
2. Brush 4 cups of a muffin tin with 1 Tbsp of coconut oil.
3. Remove the crusts from the bread. With a rolling pin, press the bread to ¼ inch thickness.
4. Brush the bread with the remaining 2 Tbsp of coconut oil, and press the bread into the prepared muffin cups to create a bowl.
5. Carefully crack an egg into each cup.
6. Top each egg evenly with tomato, cheese, basil, salt, and pepper.
7. Bake for 20 minutes.
8. Use the tip of a knife to loosen the cups from the edges of the pan.
9. Serve.

Vegetable Omelet with Goat Cheese

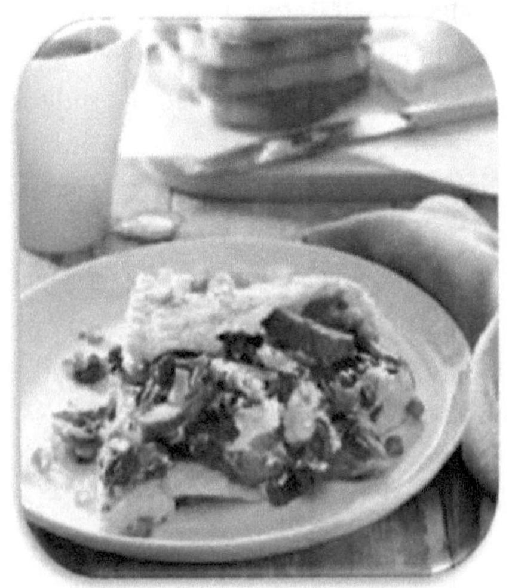

Prep time: 15 minutes
Cooking time: 20 minutes
Servings: 2

Nutrients per serving:

Carbohydrates – 12.5 g
Fat – 23.1 g
Protein – 27.4 g
Calories – 357

Ingredients:

- 1 Tbsp avocado oil
- 3 cups chopped fresh mushrooms
- 2 cups chopped fresh baby spinach
- ½ cup chopped roasted red peppers
- ½ cup chopped onion
- 1 tsp Italian seasoning
- ½ tsp salt, divided
- ½ tsp freshly ground black pepper, divided
- 5 eggs, lightly beaten
- 2 oz crumbled goat cheese

Instructions:

1. Heat the oil in a skillet.
2. Add mushrooms, spinach, red peppers, onion, Italian seasoning, and ¼ tsp each of salt and pepper.
3. Sauté the mixture for 5 minutes or until tender. Keep the mixture warm.
4. Whisk together the eggs and remaining ¼ tsp each of salt and pepper. Add to skillet. Tilt the pan to coat evenly with the egg.
5. Cook for 1 minute. Use a spatula to lift edges and allow uncooked egg to flow underneath. Cook for 2 more minutes.
6. Sprinkle goat cheese on top of the egg; spread the vegetable mixture over the goat cheese.
7. Fold the omelet in half and cook for 1 more minute or until cheese softens and egg is cooked through.

Eggs Poached in Spiced Tomato Sauce

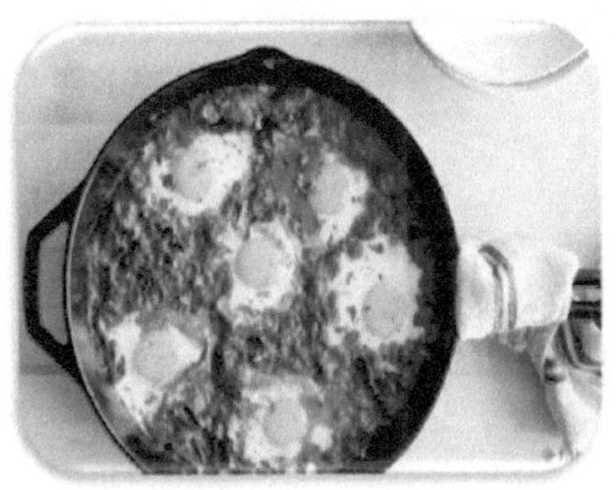

Prep time: 10 minutes
Cooking time: 15 minutes
Servings: 2

Nutrients per serving:

Carbohydrates – 34.5 g
Fat – 8.7 g
Protein – 12 g
Calories – 268

Ingredients:

- 2 Tbsp avocado oil
- ½ cup chopped onion
- ½ tsp ground cumin
- 2 cups marinara sauce
- 4 eggs
- ¼ tsp salt
- ¼ tsp freshly ground black pepper
- 4 slices frozen sprouted-grain bread, thawed and toasted

Instructions:

1. In a deep skillet, heat the oil.
2. Add the onion and cumin. Cook, stirring occasionally, for 5 minutes.
3. Add the marinara sauce. Cook for 5 minutes until gently bubbling.
4. Crack the eggs into the sauce.

5. Season with salt and pepper.
6. Cover and cook for 5 to 8 minutes.
7. Spoon 1 egg and some of the sauce onto each piece of toast. Serve.

Spinach-Red Pepper Frittata with Feta

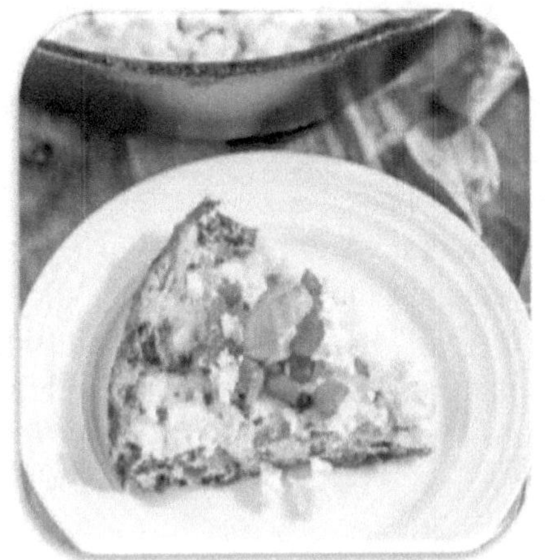

Prep time: 10 minutes
Cooking time: 10 minutes
Servings: 6

Nutrients per serving:

Carbohydrates – 2.2 g
Fat – 7.6 g
Protein – 9.7 g
Calories – 165

Ingredients:

- 2 Tbsp coconut oil
- 3 cups firmly packed fresh baby spinach
- 1 garlic clove, minced
- 8 eggs
- ½ tsp salt
- ½ tsp freshly ground black pepper
- ¼ tsp freshly ground nutmeg
- 2 jarred roasted red peppers, thinly sliced
- ½ cup crumbled feta cheese
- 2 Tbsp chopped fresh basil

Instructions:

1. In a 10-inch nonstick skillet, heat the coconut oil over medium heat.
2. Add the spinach and garlic and cook, stirring occasionally, for 2 minutes, or until the spinach is wilted.
3. In a bowl, mix the eggs, salt, pepper, and nutmeg.
4. Pour the mixture over the spinach in the skillet.
5. Top evenly with peppers and cheese.
6. Using a spatula, carefully lift the edges to let the uncooked egg flow underneath. Continue this process until the frittata is almost set.
7. Cover and cook for 2 more minutes, or until frittata is set.
8. Serve the frittata cut into wedges and top with basil.

Delightful Cinnamon and Cherry Rice Breakfast Bowl

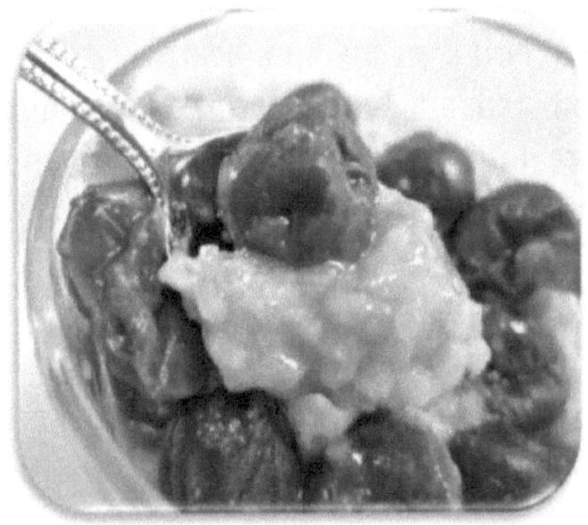

Prep time: 20 minutes
Cooking time: none
Servings: 4

Nutrients per serving:

Carbohydrates – 47 g
Fat – 5 g
Protein – 5 g
Calories – 250

Ingredients:

- 1 Tbsp olive oil
- 1 cup brown rice
- 2½ tsp cinnamon
- 1 tsp orange zest
- 1/3 cup almond milk
- ½ tsp sea salt
- 5 tsp maple syrup
- ½ tsp vanilla
- 1 tsp honey
- 1 cup dark cherries

Instructions:

1. Cook the rice.
2. Stir in the olive oil, cinnamon, salt, and orange zest.

3. Divide this mixture into four servings.
4. Pour the almond milk and the maple syrup into a saucepan and allow them to boil over medium heat.
5. Remove from heat and add the honey and vanilla.
6. Pour this sweet mixture over the rice bowls, and enjoy the healthful breakfast creation.

Hash Brown Scramble

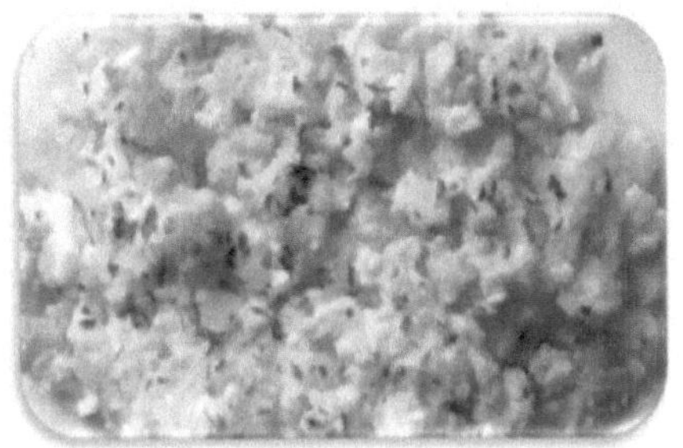

Prep time: 10 minutes
Cooking time: 20 minutes
Servings: 4

Nutrients per serving:

Carbohydrates – 11.8 g
Fat – 9.8 g
Protein – 11.9 g
Calories – 180

Ingredients:

- 4 slices natural, uncured bacon
- 6 eggs, beaten
- ½ tsp salt
- ½ tsp freshly ground black pepper
- 1 Tbsp avocado oil
- 2 cups frozen hash browns
- ½ cup chopped onion
- 1 cup chopped tomatoes

Instructions:

1. In a skillet, cook the bacon for about 5-6 minutes.
2. Remove the bacon and drain it on paper towels, reserving 2 Tbsp of drippings in pan. Crumble the bacon, and set aside.
3. Add the eggs, salt, and pepper to the skillet. Cook for 3 minutes, stirring to scramble. Remove the eggs from the skillet.
4. Heat the oil in the skillet; add the hash browns and onion. Sauté for 12 minutes, or until the hash browns are browned and the onion is

tender.

5. Stir in the bacon, scrambled eggs, and tomato.
6. Mix the scramble gently in pan for 1 minute, just enough to cook the tomatoes slightly and warm up the eggs. Serve.

LUNCH

Cottage Cheese with Raspberries and Almonds

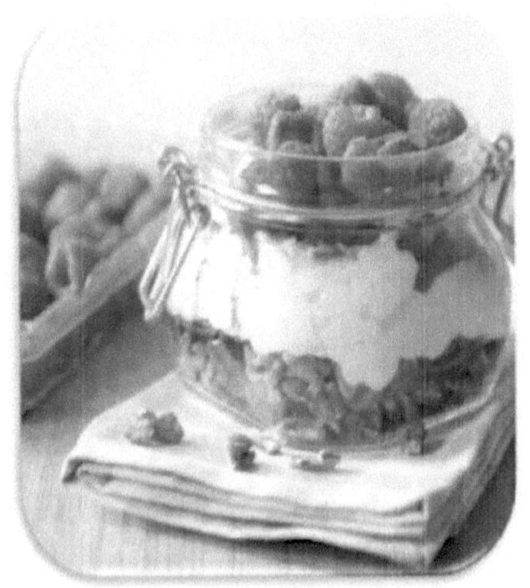

Prep time: 10 minutes
Cooking time: none
Servings: 1

Nutrients per serving:

Carbohydrates – 16 g
Fat – 14 g
Protein – 21 g
Calories – 270

Ingredients:

- ½ cup cottage cheese
- ¼ cup almonds
- ½ cup raspberries

Instructions:

1. Layer ingredients in a small bowl and serve right away.

Green Arugula and Sunflower Seed Quick Salad

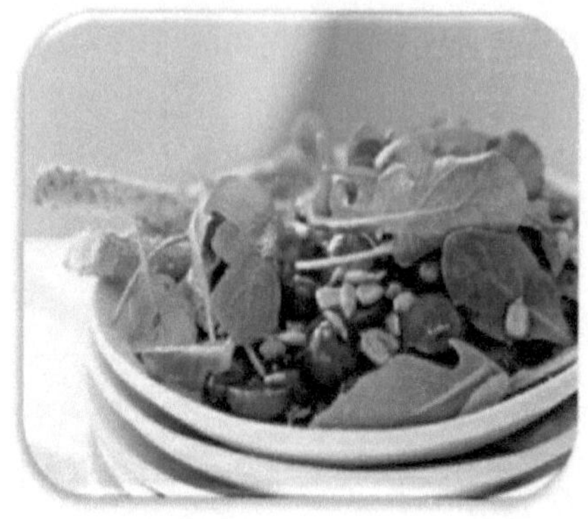

Prep time: 15 minutes
Cooking time: none
Servings: 6

Nutrients per serving:

Carbohydrates – 16 g
Fat – 14 g
Protein – 21 g
Calories – 270

Ingredients:

- 1½ tsp honey
- 4 Tbsp red wine vinegar
- 2 tsp grapeseed oil
- 1 tsp mustard
- 1 tsp maple syrup
- 2½ cups halved red grapes
- 8 cups arugula
- 2 tsp diced thyme
- 3 Tbsp toasted sunflower seeds
- ½ tsp pepper

Instructions:

1. Mix together the honey, maple syrup, vinegar, and the mustard in a medium-sized bowl.

2. Add the grapeseed oil, just a bit at a time. Stir well as you pour.
3. Mix together the grapes, arugula, thyme, and seeds in a large mixing
    bowl.
4. Add the dressing over top, and add salt and pepper.
5. Toss the salad, and enjoy.

Sizzling Tenderloins with Red Wine Vinegar and Onion

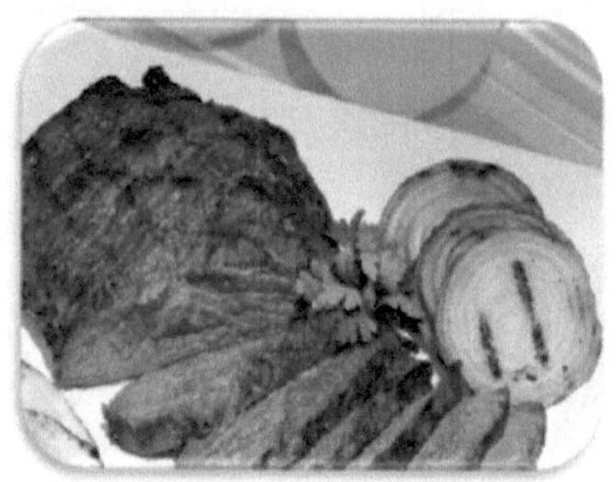

Prep time: 15 minutes
Cooking time: 20 minutes
Servings: 5

Nutrients per serving:

Carbohydrates – 12 g
Fat – 11 g
Protein – 32 g
Calories – 290

Ingredients:

- 5 (4-oz) beef tenderloins
- 1 red onion, separated into onion "rings"
- 1 tsp olive oil
- 2½ Tbsp honey
- 2½ Tbsp red wine vinegar
- 1½ tsp thyme
- ½ tsp salt

Instructions:

1. Preheat your oven's broiler.
2. Put a skillet on your stovetop over medium-high heat. Pour the olive oil into the skillet and add the onion. Cook for three minutes.
3. Pour the vinegar, honey, and the salt into the skillet. Lower the heat, and simmer 10 minutes. Stir every two minutes.
4. Season the beef with the pepper, salt, and thyme.

5. Place beef in the broiler pan, and broil for 5 minutes on each side.
6. Serve the beef steaks with the skillet ingredients, and enjoy!

Parsley Baked Sweet Potatoes

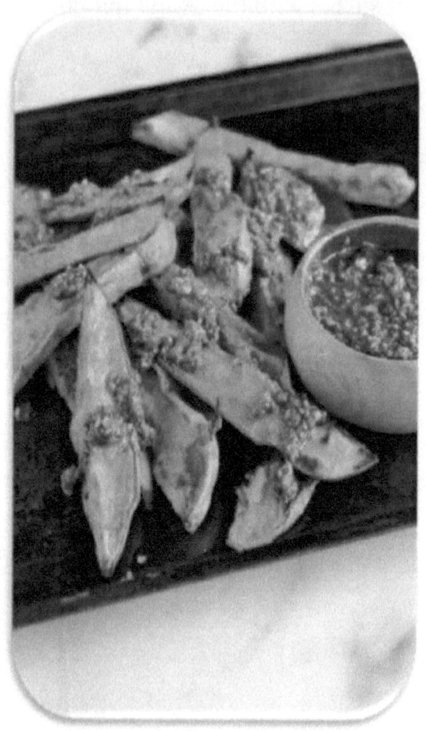

Prep time: 15 minutes
Cooking time: 32 minutes
Servings: 8

Nutrients per serving:

Carbohydrates – 34 g
Fat – 2 g
Protein – 2 g
Calories – 165

Ingredients:

- 4 peeled and sliced sweet potatoes
- ½ tsp salt
- ½ tsp pepper
- 1½ Tbsp olive oil
- 1½ Tbsp diced parsley
- 2 minced garlic cloves

- 2 tsp orange zest

Instructions:

1. Preheat the oven to 400° F.
2. Combine the sliced sweet potatoes, olive oil, salt, and pepper together in a medium-sized mixing bowl.
3. Toss the potatoes and then position them on a baking sheet.
4. Bake them for 32 minutes, making sure to flip them halfway through.
5. Mix together orange zest, parsley, and the minced garlic in a small mixing bowl. Sprinkle this mixture over the just-out-of-the-oven sweet potatoes slices, and enjoy!

Corn and Potato Chowder

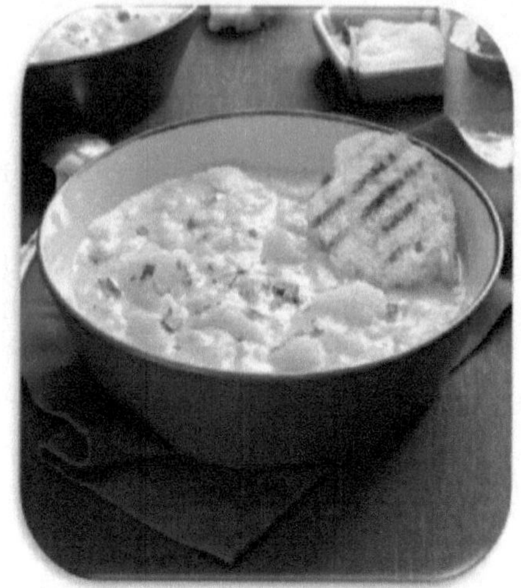

Prep time: 10 minutes
Cooking time: 20 minutes
Servings: 4

Nutrients per serving:

Carbohydrates – 25.5 g
Fat – 12.1 g
Protein – 7.1 g
Calories – 230

Ingredients:

- 2 Tbsp avocado oil
- ½ cup chopped onion
- 1½ cups fresh corn kernels (about 3 ears of corn)
- 1 cup milk
- 1 (14.5-oz) can reduced-sodium vegetable broth
- ½ lb new potatoes, diced
- ½ tsp salt
- ½ tsp freshly ground black pepper

Instructions:

1. Heat the oil in a Dutch oven.

2. Add the onion and corn and cook, stirring frequently, for 5 minutes, or until the onion and corn are tender.
3. Add remaining ingredients and bring to a boil. Then simmer for 15 minutes.
4. Mash the mixture with a potato masher to reach the desired consistency.
5. Serve hot.

Tuna-Barley Salad with Roasted Red Peppers and Artichokes

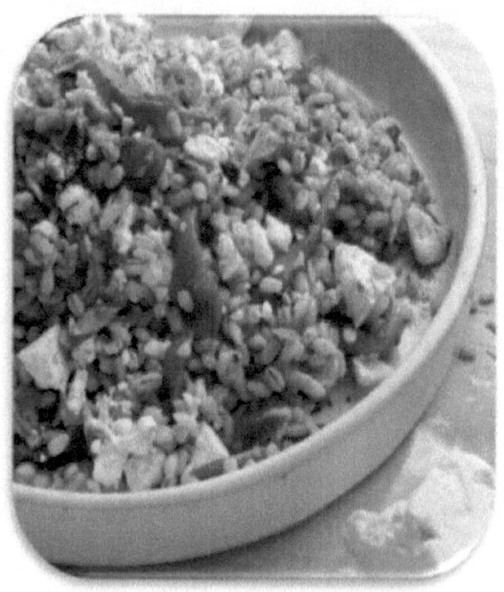

Prep time: 10 minutes
Cooking time: 20 minutes
Servings: 4

Nutrients per serving:

Carbohydrates – 63.5 g
Fat – 13 g
Protein – 30.2 g
Calories – 429

Ingredients:

- 1½ cups uncooked barley
- 1 (12-oz) jar artichoke hearts, drained, chopped
- 1 (12-oz) jar roasted red peppers, drained, chopped
- 3 cups chopped fresh baby spinach
- 2 (5-oz) cans albacore tuna in water, drained, flaked
- 3 Tbsp extra-virgin olive oil
- 2 Tbsp lemon juice
- 1 Tbsp chopped fresh basil
- ½ tsp salt
- ½ tsp freshly ground black pepper

Instructions:

1. Cook the barley then drain. Rinse under cold water to cool.
2. In a large bowl, combine the barley, artichokes, peppers, spinach, and tuna.
3. In a separate bowl, whisk together the oil, lemon juice, basil, salt, and pepper.
4. Pour the dressing over the barley mixture. Toss gently to coat and serve.

Creamy Asparagus Soup

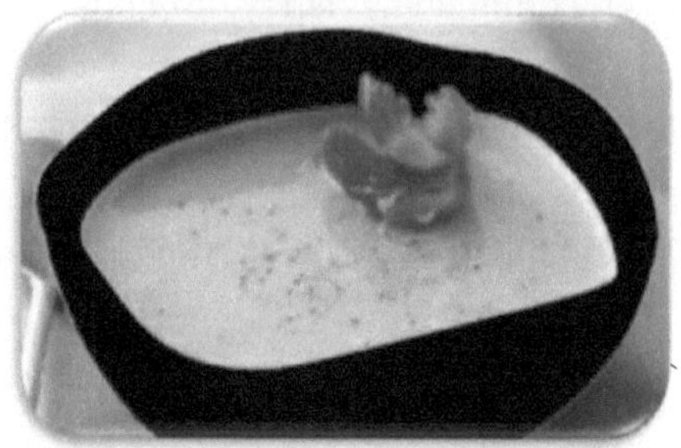

Prep time: 15 minutes
Cooking time: 15 minutes
Servings: 4

Nutrients per serving:

Carbohydrates – 12 g
Fat – 3.8 g
Protein – 12.4 g
Calories – 122

Ingredients:

- 2 Tbsp avocado oil
- 2 garlic cloves, minced
- 2 lbs fresh asparagus, coarsely chopped
- 4 cups reduced-sodium vegetable broth
- ½ cup plain Greek yogurt
- ½ tsp salt
- ½ tsp freshly ground black pepper

Instructions:

1. In a Dutch oven, heat the oil.
2. Add the garlic and asparagus and sauté for 3 minutes.
3. Add the broth; cover and cook for 5 minutes or until the asparagus is tender.
4. Process the soup in a blender or until smooth.
5. Return the soup to the Dutch oven. Stir in the yogurt, salt, and pepper.
6. Cook over medium heat for 5 minutes. Serve hot.

Almond Butter-Apple Sandwiches

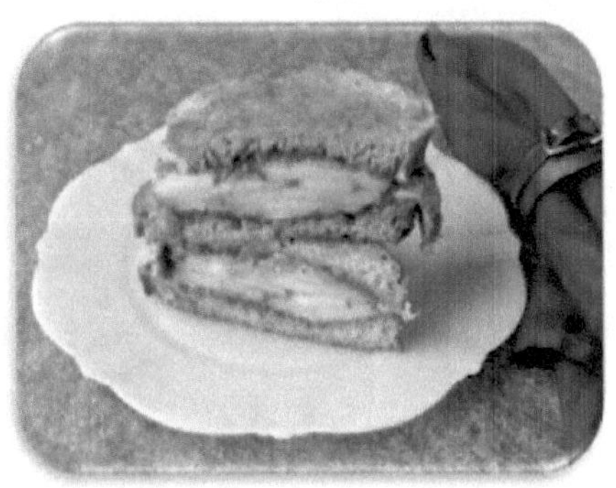

Prep time: 10 minutes
Cooking time: none
Servings: 4

Nutrients per serving:

Carbohydrates – 59.9 g
Fat – 16.1 g
Protein – 15.1 g
Calories – 428

Ingredients:

- 8 Tbsp all-natural almond butter, divided
- 8 slices frozen sprouted-grain bread, thawed and toasted
- 1 apple, thinly sliced
- 4 Tbsp honey, divided
- 1 tsp ground cinnamon, divided

Instructions:

1. Spread 1 Tbsp of the almond butter onto one side of each slice of bread.
2. Arrange the apple slices over the almond butter in one layer on four slices of bread.
3. Drizzle 1 Tbsp of honey over the apples and sprinkle with cinnamon.
4. Top with the remaining apple butter bread slices, and serve.

Turkey-Cucumber Sandwiches with Mashed Avocado

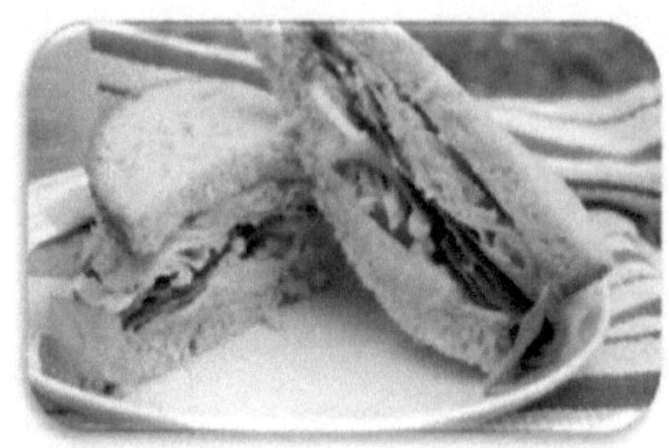

Prep time: 10 minutes
Cooking time: none
Servings: 4

Nutrients per serving:

Carbohydrates – 44.1 g
Fat – 2.1 g
Protein – 17.9 g
Calories – 321

Ingredients:

- 1 avocado, mashed
- 1 Tbsp lime juice
- ¼ tsp salt
- ¼ tsp freshly ground black pepper
- 8 slices frozen sprouted-grain bread, thawed and toasted
- 1 cucumber, thinly sliced
- ¼ cup fresh basil leaves
- 7 oz sliced natural, deli-roasted turkey (no nitrates)

Instructions:

1. Spread mashed avocado on one side of each slice of bread. Top 1 slice with spinach, turkey and onion; drizzle with lemon juice. Cover with remaining slice of bread, avocado side down.

Pasta Salad with Avocado-Pesto Cream Sauce

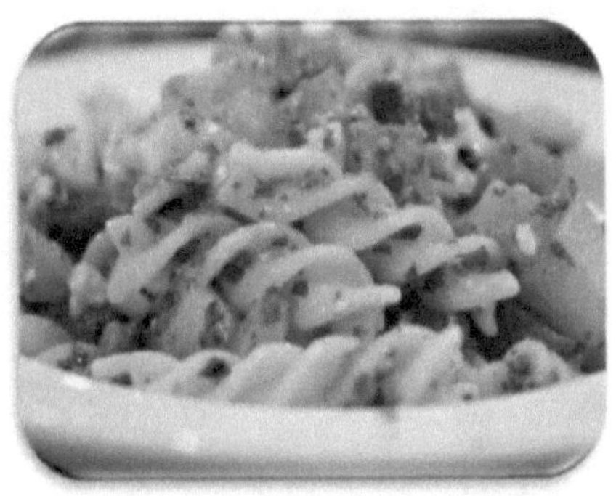

Prep time: 10 minutes
Cooking time: 20 minutes
Servings: 4

Nutrients per serving:

Carbohydrates – 64 g
Fat – 28.6 g
Protein – 19.1 g
Calories – 564

Ingredients:

- 12 oz 100% whole-wheat fusilli
- 2 avocados, coarsely chopped
- 3 Tbsp lemon juice
- 3 Tbsp pesto
- 1 Tbsp extra-virgin olive oil
- ¼ tsp salt
- 1 cup chopped tomatoes
- 1 cup fresh basil, chopped

Instructions:

1. Cook the pasta. Drain and rinse under cold water.
2. Combine lemon juice, pesto, oil, and salt.
3. In a bowl, mix the pasta, avocados, tomatoes, basil and sauce. Serve.

SNACKS

Herbed Pita Chips

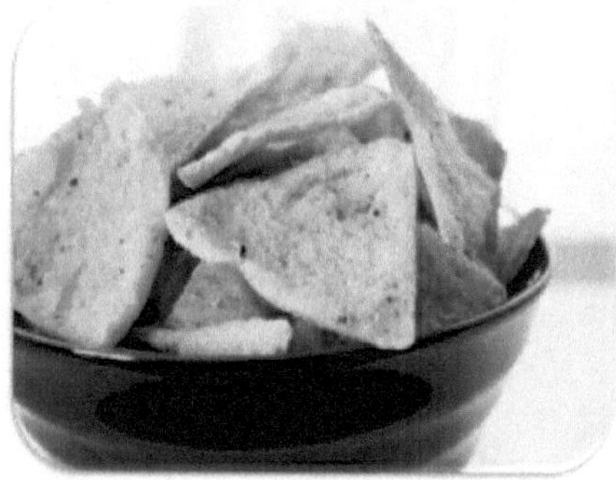

Prep time: 10 minutes
Cooking time: 20 minutes
Servings: 6

Nutrients per serving:

Carbohydrates – 21 g
Fat – 8.2 g
Protein – 4 g
Calories – 171

Ingredients:

- 4 100% whole-grain pitas
- 3 Tbsp coconut oil, melted
- 1 Tbsp Italian seasoning
- ½ tsp salt
- ½ tsp freshly ground black pepper

Instructions:

1. Preheat the oven to 400°F.
2. Cut the pitas into 6 triangles. Separate the triangles.
3. Put the pita triangles on a rimmed baking sheet and brush them with the coconut oil.
4. Sprinkle the pita triangles evenly with the Italian seasoning, salt, and pepper.
5. Bake for about 10 minutes.

6. Let the chips cool. Serve.

Crunchy Cumin-Spiced Chickpeas

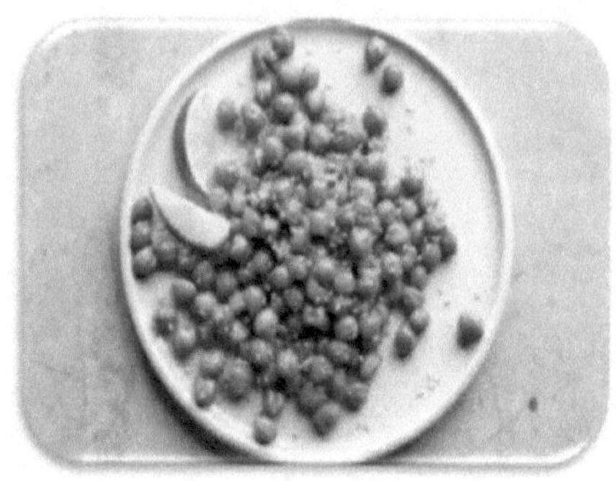

Prep time: 5 minutes
Cooking time: 40 minutes
Servings: 4

Nutrients per serving:

Carbohydrates – 38.4 g
Fat – 6 g
Protein – 12.2 g
Calories – 247

Ingredients:

- 2 (15.5-oz) cans chickpeas, drained, rinsed, and dried
- 2 Tbsp coconut oil
- 2 tsp ground cumin
- 1 tsp garlic powder
- ½ tsp salt

Instructions:

1. Preheat the oven to 400°F.
2. Line a baking sheet with parchment paper.
3. In a large bowl, combine the chickpeas, coconut oil, cumin, garlic powder, and salt.
4. Spread the chickpeas into one layer on the prepared baking sheet.
5. Bake for 45 minutes, turning occasionally, until the chickpeas are lightly browned and crispy.
6. Serve hot.

Zucchini-Based Hummus

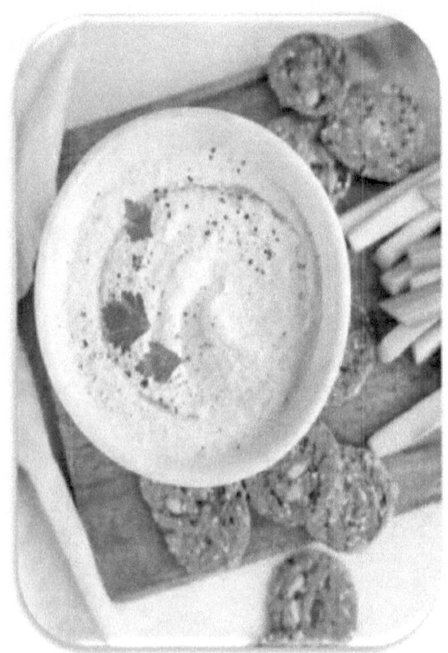

Prep time: 15 minutes
Cooking time: none
Servings: 10

Nutrients per serving:

Carbohydrates – 3.5 g
Fat – 11 g
Protein – 2 g
Calories – 130

Ingredients:

- 2 peeled and chopped zucchinis
- ½ cup lemon juice
- 1/3 cup tahini
- 2 tsp cumin
- ½ cup olive oil
- 4 minced garlic cloves
- Salt and pepper, to taste

Instructions:

1. In a food processor, blend all ingredients. Note that you can always add extra tahini to make a thicker paste.
2. Serve the hummus with carrots, broccoli, celery sticks, or cucumber, and enjoy!

Baked Tortilla Chips

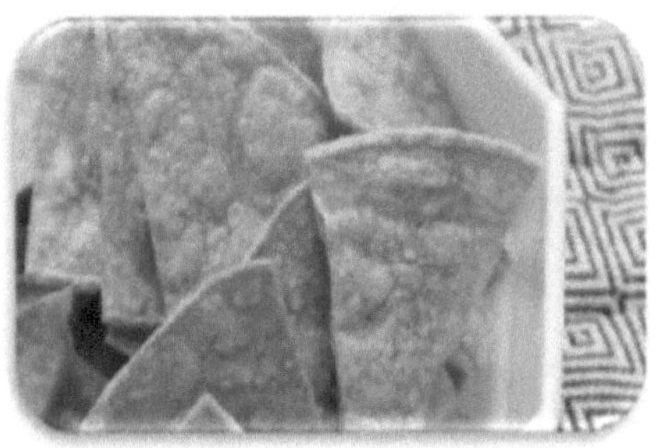

Prep time: 10 minutes
Cooking time: 10 minutes
Servings: 8

Nutrients per serving:

Carbohydrates – 18 g
Fat – 5.3 g
Protein – 3.8 g
Calories – 127

Ingredients:

- 2 Tbsp coconut oil, for greasing
- 6 (8-inch) 100% whole-wheat tortillas
- ¼ tsp salt

Instructions:

1. Preheat the oven to 425°F.
2. Coat a baking sheet with coconut oil.
3. Cut each tortilla into 8 wedges.
4. Brush the wedges evenly with the coconut oil and sprinkle with salt.
5. Arrange tortillas in one layer on the prepared baking sheet. Bake for 8 minutes or until crisp.
6. Let the chips cool. Serve.

Pesto Essential Goat Cheese Spread

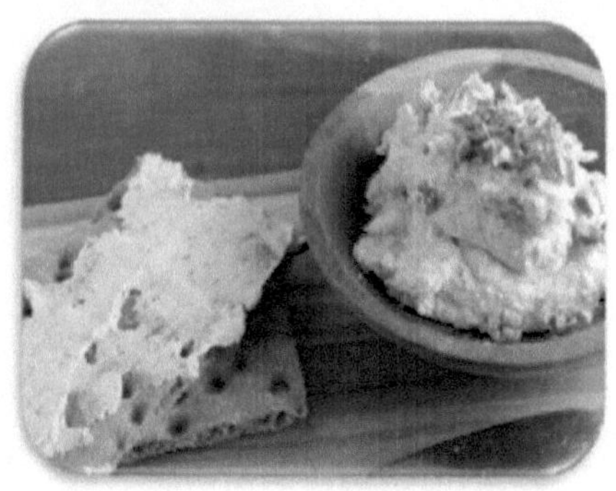

Prep time: 15 minutes
Cooking time: none
Servings: 8

Nutrients per serving:

Carbohydrates – 1 g
Fat – 16 g
Protein – 9 g
Calories – 190

Ingredients:

- 10 oz softened goat cheese
- 3 minced garlic cloves
- 2½ cups basil leaves
- 2½ Tbsp olive oil
- 1/3 cup diced pecans
- Salt and pepper, to taste

Instructions:

1. Blend the goat cheese, garlic, basil, and the pecans together in a food processor, slowly adding the olive oil.
2. Once you've created a creamy consistency, season with pepper and salt. Serve with artisan, whole-grain bread for a mid-day snack.

Garlic-Herb Popcorn

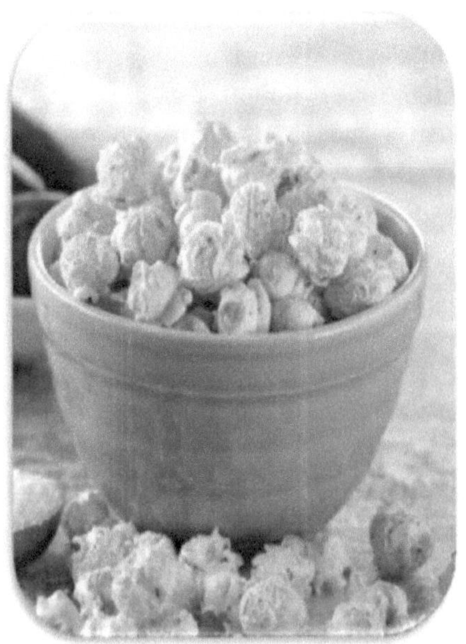

Prep time: 5 minutes
Cooking time: 10 minutes
Servings: 4

Nutrients per serving:

Carbohydrates – 2.5 g
Fat – 6.1 g
Protein – 0.4 g
Calories – 81

Ingredients:

- 2 Tbsp coconut oil
- ½ cup organic popcorn kernels
- 1 Tbsp garlic powder
- 1 Tbsp Italian seasoning
- ½ tsp salt

Instructions:

1. In a pot over high heat, add the oil and popcorn kernels.
2. Cook, covered, swirling the pan occasionally, until the popcorn

begins to pop slowly.
3. Keep it covered after removing from the heat until the popcorn finishes popping.
4. Add the garlic powder, Italian seasoning, and salt to the popcorn, tossing to coat. Serve.

Salt and Pepper Kale Chips

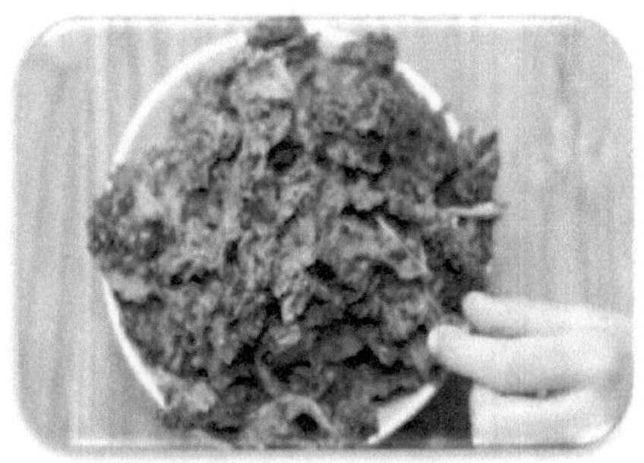

Prep time: 10 minutes
Cooking time: 15 minutes
Servings: 8

Nutrients per serving:

Carbohydrates – 6.2 g
Fat – 0.4 g
Protein – 1.7 g
Calories – 33

Ingredients:

- 2 Tbsp avocado oil, plus additional for greasing
- 1 lb kale
- ½ tsp salt
- ½ tsp freshly ground black pepper

Instructions:

1. Preheat the oven to 350°F.
2. Brush two rimmed baking sheets with oil.
3. Remove the center rib and stems from the kale; tear the leaves into 2-inch pieces.
4. Place the kale in a bowl and add 2 Tbsp of oil, salt, and pepper. Toss well to coat.
5. Arrange the kale in a layer on the baking sheets.
6. Bake for about 15 minutes.
7. Let cool. Serve or store in an airtight container.

Tabbouleh

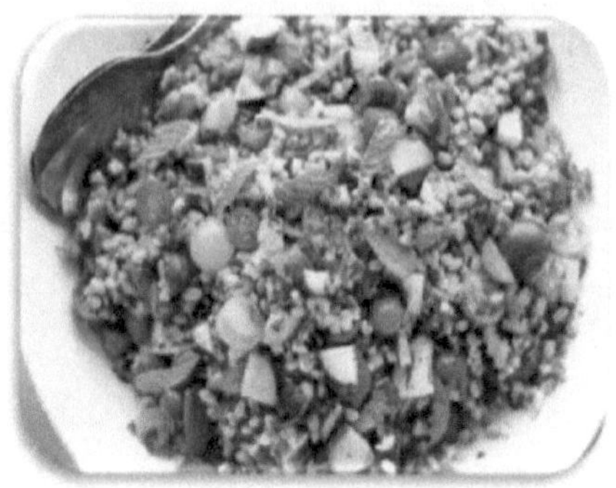

Prep time: 10 minutes
Cooking time: none
Servings: 6

Nutrients per serving:

Carbohydrates – 15 g
Fat – 7.5 g
Protein – 2.8 g
Calories – 127

Ingredients:

- ½ cup bulgur wheat
- 3 Tbsp extra-virgin olive oil
- 1 cup chopped fresh parsley
- ½ cup chopped fresh mint
- 2 tomatoes, chopped
- 1 small cucumber, peeled and finely chopped
- ¼ cup finely chopped red onion
- Juice and zest of 1 lemon
- ½ tsp salt
- ½ tsp freshly ground black pepper

Instructions:

1. Cook the bulgur wheat. Drain and rinse under cold water.
2. In a large bowl, combine all ingredients. Serve.

Slow Cooker Apple Sauce

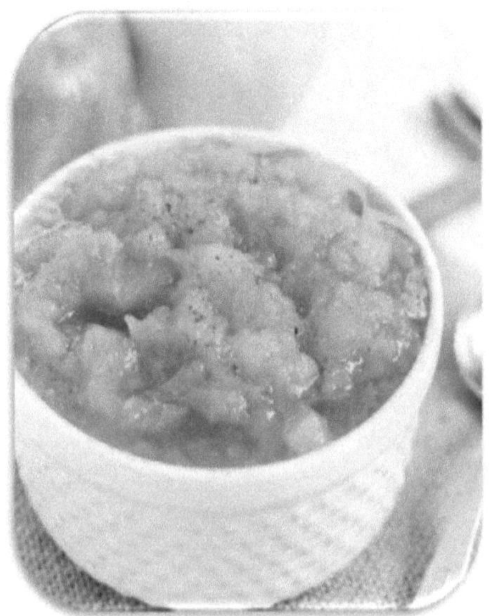

Prep time: 10 minutes
Cooking time: 6 hours
Servings: 3

Nutrients per serving:

Carbohydrates – 17.1 g
Fat – 0 g
Protein – 0 g
Calories – 65

Ingredients:

- 8 apples, peeled, cored, cut into wedges
- 1 Tbsp lemon juice
- 1 Tbsp evaporated cane juice

Instructions:

1. Combine all ingredients in a 4- to 5-quart slow cooker.
2. Cover and cook on low for 6 hours. Stir occasionally.
3. Transfer the applesauce to a blender or food processor and pulse to desired consistency.

Chocolate-Almond Dip with Strawberries

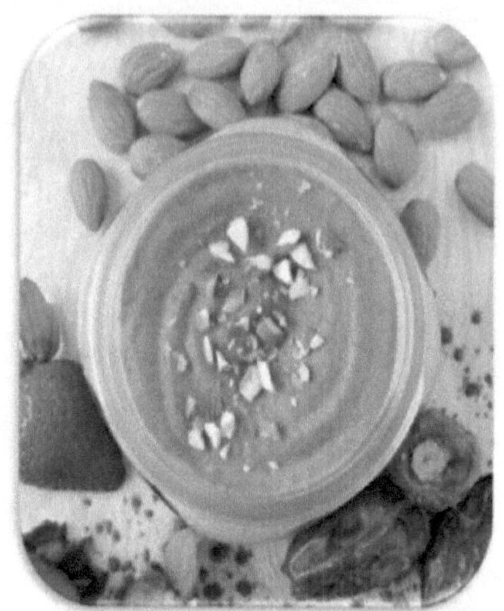

Prep time: 10 minutes
Cooking time: none
Servings: 2

Nutrients per serving:

Carbohydrates – 4.8 g
Fat – 4.6 g
Protein – 2.3 g
Calories – 67

Ingredients:

- ½ cup all-natural almond butter
- ½ cup plain Greek yogurt
- 1 oz 70% bittersweet chocolate, melted
- ¼ cup milk
- 2 Tbsp flaxseed
- 1 quart fresh strawberries
- ¼ cup chopped almonds

Instructions:

1. Stir together the almond butter, yogurt, chocolate, milk, and

flaxseed.
2. Serve topped with almonds and strawberries.

VEGETARIAN DINNER
Vegetarian Chili

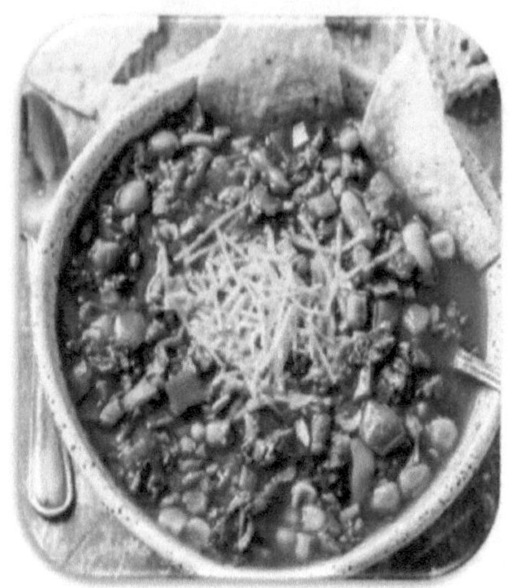

Prep time: 5 minutes
Cooking time: 40 minutes
Servings: 4

Nutrients per serving:

Carbohydrates – 156.5 g
Fat – 3.9 g
Protein – 56.1 g
Calories – 920

Ingredients:

- 2 Tbsp avocado oil
- 1 onion, chopped
- 1 green bell pepper, chopped
- 2 garlic cloves, minced
- 2 tsp ground cumin
- 1 tsp smoked paprika
- ½ tsp red pepper flakes
- 1 (14.5-oz) can reduced-sodium vegetable broth
- 1 cup diced sweet potato
- 1 (28-oz) can whole tomatoes, chopped

- 1 (15-oz) can pinto beans, drained and rinsed
- 1 (15-oz) can kidney beans, drained and rinsed
- ½ cup shredded sharp white Cheddar cheese
- 2 Tbsp chopped fresh cilantro leaves, for garnish

Instructions:

1. In a Dutch oven, heat the oil.
2. Add the onion and bell pepper. Cook for 5 minutes or until tender.
3. Stir in the garlic, cumin, paprika, and red pepper flakes. Cook for 2 more minutes.
4. Add the vegetable broth, sweet potato, tomatoes, pinto beans, and kidney beans. Bring the mixture to a boil.
5. Reduce the heat, simmer for 30 minutes or until the sweet potato is tender and the chili is thickened, stirring occasionally.
6. Serve the chili topped with cheese and garnished with cilantro.

Grilled Mini Veggie Pizzas

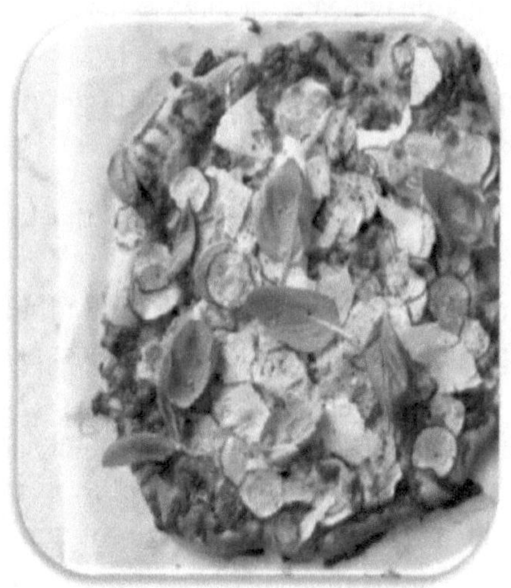

Prep time: 15 minutes
Cooking time: 5 minutes
Servings: 4

Nutrients per serving:

Carbohydrates – 27.8 g
Fat – 13.2 g
Protein – 11.2 g
Calories – 275

Ingredients:

- 4 100% whole-grain tortillas
- 1 cup marinara sauce
- 2 cups sliced zucchini and yellow squash
- ½ cup sliced red onion
- ½ cup pitted, halved Kalamata olives
- ½ cup crumbled feta cheese
- ½ cup shredded white Cheddar cheese

Instructions:

1. Preheat the grill to medium heat.
2. Spread each tortilla with ¼ cup of marinara sauce, then top evenly

with the zucchini, yellow squash, onion, olives, and cheeses.
3. Cover the grill with the grill lid and cook for 2 to 3 minutes.
4. Slice and serve.

Mushroom Barley Risotto

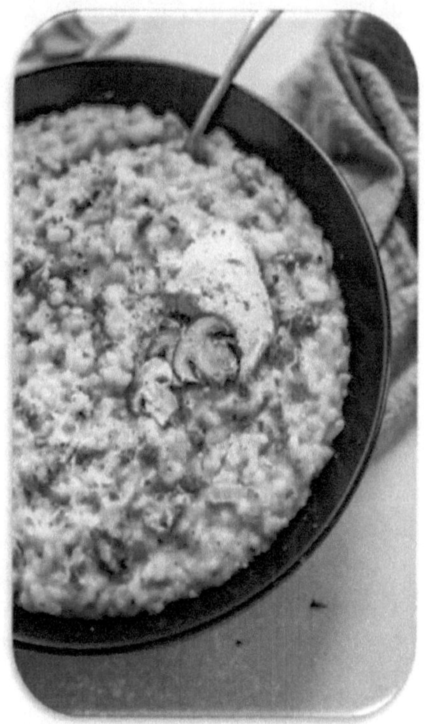

Prep time: 10 minutes
Cooking time: 35 minutes
Servings: 4

Nutrients per serving:

Carbohydrates – 78.5 g
Fat – 11.4 g
Protein – 31.1 g
Calories – 524

Ingredients:

- 6 cups reduced-sodium vegetable broth
- 2 Tbsp avocado oil
- 3 garlic cloves, minced
- ½ cup chopped onion
- 1 lb portobello mushrooms, chopped
- 2 cups uncooked pearled barley

- ½ tsp dried thyme
- ½ tsp salt
- ½ tsp freshly ground black pepper
- 1 cup freshly grated Parmesan cheese

Instructions:

1. In a saucepan, heat the broth. Keep warm.
2. In a Dutch oven, heat the oil.
3. Add the garlic and onion. Cook for 5 minutes.
4. Add the mushrooms. Cook for 5 more minutes.
5. Stir in the barley. Cook for 1 minute or until toasted.
6. Stir in the thyme and 1 cup of the hot broth. Cook for 3 minutes, or until nearly all the broth has evaporated.
7. Stir in the salt, pepper, and ¾ cup of broth. Cook until the broth is nearly all evaporated.
8. Continue adding more broth ½ cup at a time, until the barley is tender and the risotto is creamy, 18 to 20 minutes.
9. Stir in the cheese just before serving.

Chinese Cashew Chicken

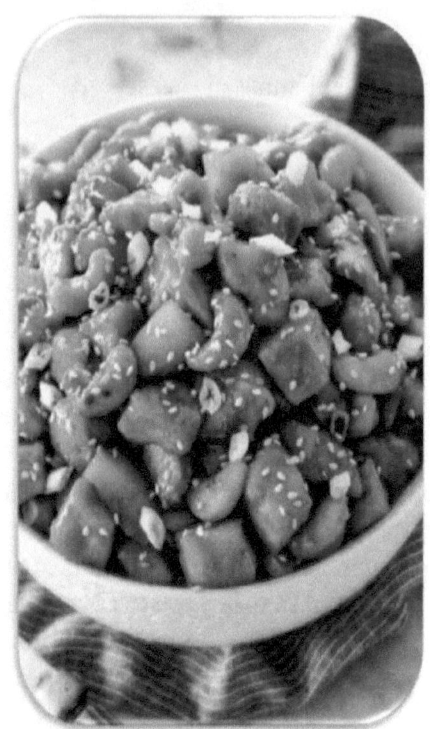

Prep time: 15 minutes
Cooking time: 12 minutes
Servings: 4

Nutrients per serving:

Carbohydrates – 67 g
Fat – 11 g
Protein – 16 g
Calories – 430

Ingredients:

- 5 oz sliced chicken breast
- 1¼ cup frozen peas
- 2½ Tbsp olive oil
- 1/3 cup soy sauce
- 1 cup sliced and roasted red peppers
- ¾ cup diced pineapple

- 5 cups pre-cooked brown rice
- Juice from 1 lemon
- ½ cup cashews
- ½ tsp pepper

Instructions:

1. Pour olive oil into a saucepan and sauté the chicken strips over medium-high until they are golden brown.
2. Add the frozen peas and cook for 8 minutes.
3. Add the peppers and pineapple and cook for an additional 4 minutes, stirring occasionally.
4. Add the pre-cooked brown rice and stir well.
5. Season with the lemon juice, soy sauce, and pepper, and then add the cashews. Stir well, and enjoy.

Rice Noodles with Ginger Salmon

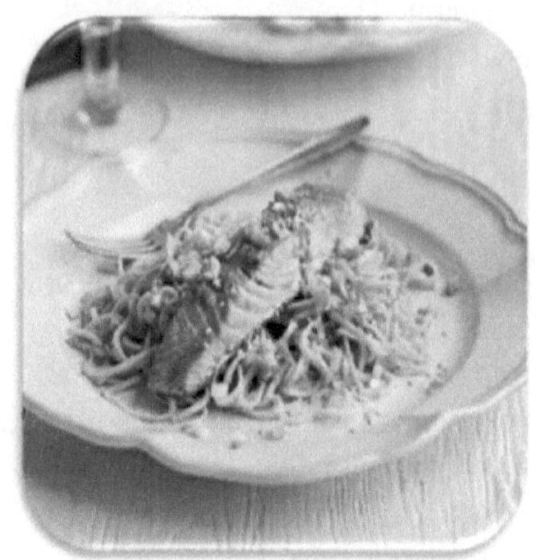

Prep time: 15 minutes
Cooking time: 12 minutes
Servings: 4

Nutrients per serving:

Carbohydrates – 1 g
Fat – 20 g
Protein – 13 g
Calories – 250

Ingredients:

- 16 oz salmon (or 2 8-oz salmon steaks)
- 3 Tbsp olive oil
- 5 oz brown rice noodles, cooked according to package instructions
- ½ tsp salt
- 1½ Tbsp sesame oil
- 1 Tbsp grated ginger
- 2 Tbsp diced mint
- 3 Tbsp coconut milk

Instructions:

1. Preheat the broiler.
2. Brush salmon with the oil, and season with salt and pepper.

3. Place salmon on a baking sheet and broil for five minutes on each side. The fish should flake.
4. In a saucepan over on low heat, mix together the precooked brown rice noodles, sesame oil, coconut milk, and the mint leaves. Stir well until warm.
5. On a plate, layer the salmon over the noodles and serve.

Creole Red Beans and Rice

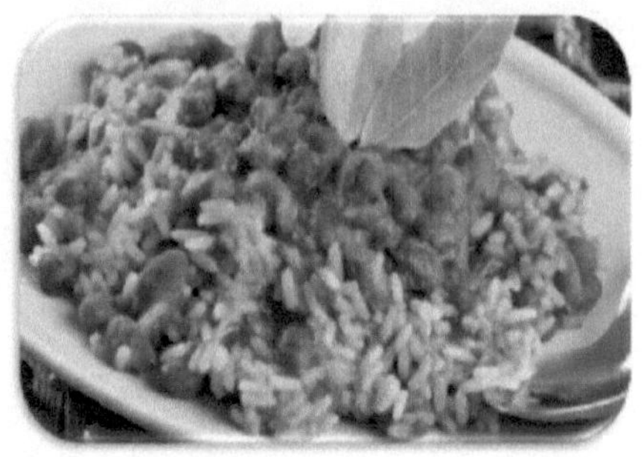

Prep time: 10 minutes
Cooking time: 1 hour
Servings: 4

Nutrients per serving:

Carbohydrates – 194.1 g
Fat – 11.9 g
Protein – 56.6 g
Calories – 1089

Ingredients:

- 1½ cups uncooked brown rice
- 2 Tbsp coconut oil
- 1 (8-oz) package pre-chopped onion, celery, and bell pepper
- 3 garlic cloves, minced
- 2 (15-oz) cans red beans, drained and rinsed
- 1 (14.5-oz) can diced tomatoes
- 1 (14.5-oz) can reduced-sodium vegetable broth
- 1 tsp dried thyme
- 1 tsp dried oregano
- 1 tsp smoked paprika
- ¾ tsp salt
- ½ tsp freshly ground black pepper
- ½ tsp cayenne pepper
- Hot sauce (optional)

Instructions:

1. Prepare rice; keep warm.
2. In a Dutch oven, heat the oil.
3. Add the onion, celery, and bell pepper mix. Cook for 5 minutes or until the vegetables are tender.
4. Add the garlic. Cook for another 2 minutes.
5. Mash one can of beans. Add the mashed beans, remaining can of beans, tomatoes, broth, thyme, oregano, paprika, salt, pepper, and cayenne pepper to the Dutch oven.
6. Bring to a boil. Simmer on low for 30 minutes.
7. Serve the Creole red beans over rice with hot sauce.

Curried Chickpeas with Spinach and Brown Rice

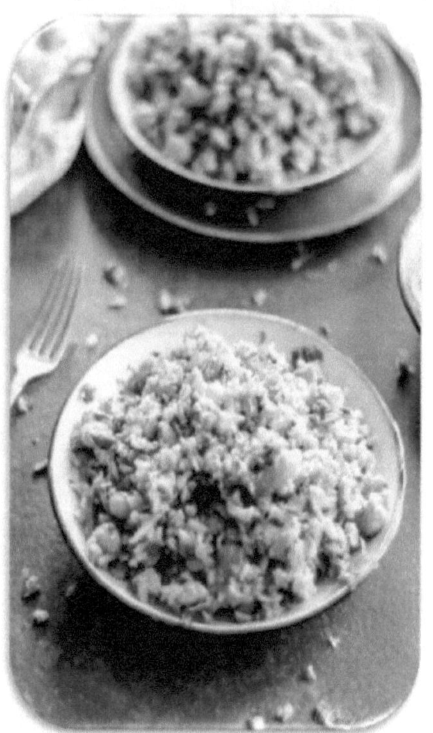

Prep time: 5 minutes
Cooking time: 40 minutes
Servings: 4

Nutrients per serving:

Carbohydrates – 170.3 g
Fat – 21.8 g
Protein – 48 g
Calories – 1039

Ingredients:

- 2 cups cooked brown rice
- 2 Tbsp coconut oil
- 1 cup chopped red onion
- 2 garlic cloves, minced
- 1 Tbsp grated fresh ginger
- 2 Tbsp curry powder

- 1 (10-oz) bag fresh baby spinach
- 1 (14.5-oz) can stewed tomatoes, drained
- 1 (14.5-oz) can reduced-sodium vegetable broth
- 2 (15.5-oz) cans chickpeas, drained, rinsed
- 4 sprigs fresh basil leaves, for garnish

Instructions:

1. In a skillet, heat the coconut oil.
2. Add the onion, garlic, and ginger and sauté for 5 minutes.
3. Stir in the curry powder and cook for 1 more minute.
4. Add the spinach, tomatoes, and vegetable broth. Cook for 5 minutes.
5. Add the chickpeas. Cook for 10 more minutes.
6. Garnish with the basil and serve with the rice.

Vietnamese Tofu Lettuce Wraps

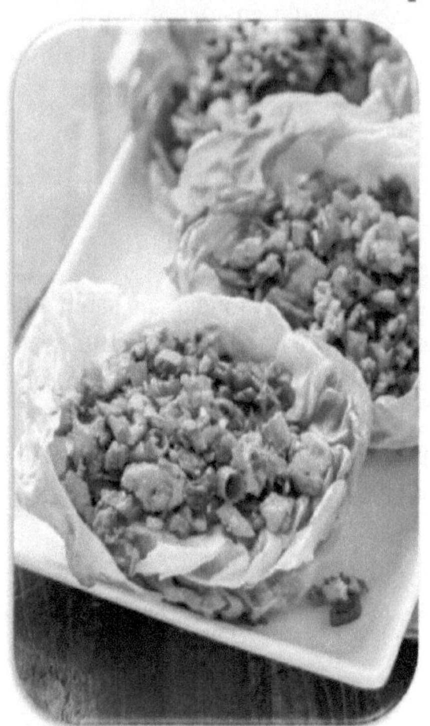

Prep time: 10 minutes
Cooking time: 10 minutes
Servings: 4

Nutrients per serving:

Carbohydrates – 35.1 g
Fat – 5.6 g
Protein – 21.3 g
Calories – 404

Ingredients:

- 1 lb extra-firm tofu, drained
- ½ cup lime juice
- ¼ cup honey
- 3 garlic cloves, minced
- 2 Tbsp fish sauce (optional)
- 2 Tbsp tamari or coconut aminos

- 1 Tbsp grated fresh ginger
- 1 tsp sambal oelek chili hot sauce
- 1 Tbsp coconut oil
- 1 head Boston lettuce, leaves separated
- ½ cup fresh cilantro leaves
- ¼ cup fresh mint leaves
- ¼ cup chopped dry-roasted peanuts
- 1 carrot, peeled and grated
- ½ cucumber, thinly sliced

Instructions:

1. Place the tofu in a baking dish.
2. In a medium bowl, whisk together the lime juice, honey, garlic, fish sauce, tamari, ginger, and hot sauce.
3. Pour the marinade over the tofu.
4. Cover and let stand for 30 minutes.
5. Remove the tofu, reserving the marinade.
6. Heat a nonstick skillet, and add the coconut oil.
7. Brown the tofu slices for 3 minutes on each side.
8. Place one tofu slice in the center of each lettuce leaf. Top with cilantro, mint, peanuts, carrot, and cucumber. Drizzle with the reserved marinade, and roll up.

Vegetable Fried Rice

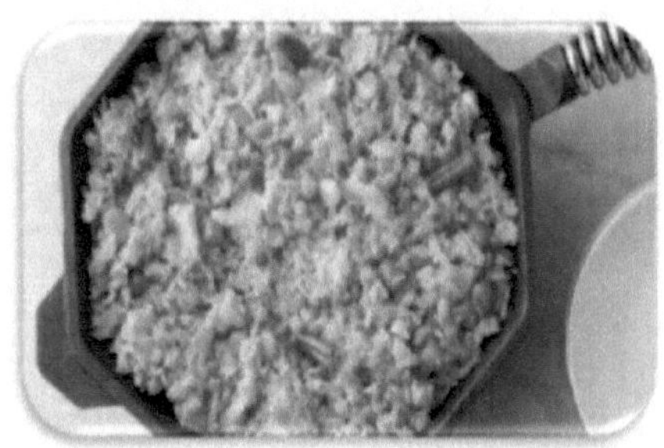

Prep time: 10 minutes
Cooking time: 1 hour
Servings: 4

Nutrients per serving:

Carbohydrates – 87.8 g
Fat – 31.6 g
Protein – 20.7 g
Calories – 709

Ingredients:

- 2½ cups brown rice, cooked
- 2 Tbsp coconut oil
- 3 eggs, lightly beaten
- 3 green onions, cut into 1-inch pieces
- 3 cups frozen mixed vegetables, thawed
- 1 red bell pepper, cut into strips
- 2 garlic cloves, minced
- 1 tsp grated fresh ginger
- 2 Tbsp brown rice vinegar
- 3 Tbsp tamari or coconut aminos
- 1 Tbsp dark sesame oil
- 1 cup unsalted cashews

Instructions:

1. In a skillet, heat 1 Tbsp of coconut oil.
2. Add the eggs, and cook for 1 minute, stirring with a spatula to scramble. Remove the egg from the pan, and keep warm.

3. Add the remaining 1 Tbsp of coconut oil to the pan.
4. Add the green onions, frozen vegetables, bell pepper, garlic, and ginger. Sauté for 5 minutes or until the vegetables are tender.
5. In a bowl, mix together the vinegar, tamari, and sesame oil.
6. Add the cooked rice to pan.
7. Stir in egg and vinegar mixture. Cook for 30 seconds or until mixture is hot, stirring constantly.
8. Top each serving with cashews.

MEAT & SEAFOOD

Spice-Rubbed Salmon with Citrus Salsa and Steamed Asparagus

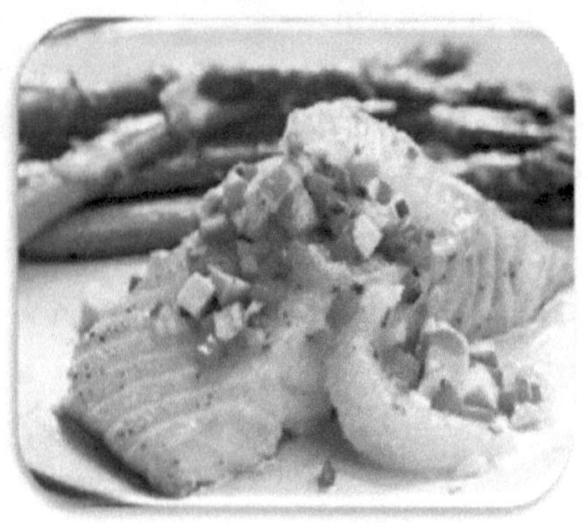

Prep time: 15 minutes
Cooking time: 10 minutes
Servings: 4

Nutrients per serving:

Carbohydrates – 21 g
Fat – 14.6 g
Protein – 38.6 g
Calories – 343

Ingredients:

- 4 skinless salmon fillets
- 1 tsp ground cumin
- 1 tsp smoked paprika
- 1 tsp salt
- 1 tsp freshly ground black pepper
- ½ lb fresh asparagus
- 2 oranges, peeled and sectioned
- 1 ruby red grapefruit, peeled and sectioned
- 1 jalapeño pepper, minced
- Juice and zest of 1 lime
- ¼ cup extra-virgin olive oil
- 3 Tbsp chopped fresh cilantro

Instructions:

1. Preheat the grill to medium-high heat.
2. Rub the salmon fillets evenly with cumin, paprika, and ½ teaspoon each of salt and pepper.
3. Place the aspagus on a large sheet of aluminum foil; sprinkle evenly with ¼ tsp each of salt and pepper. Fold the aluminum foil to create a packet.
4. Grill the salmon for 3 to 4 minutes on each side or until done.
5. Grill the asparagus for 10 minutes or until crisp-tender.
6. Chop the oranges and grapefruit and place them in a medium bowl.
7. Stir in the remaining ¼ tsp each of salt and pepper, jalapeño pepper, lime juice and zest, olive oil, and cilantro.
8. Spoon the salsa over the salmon. Serve the salmon with the asparagus on the side.

Shrimp Succotash

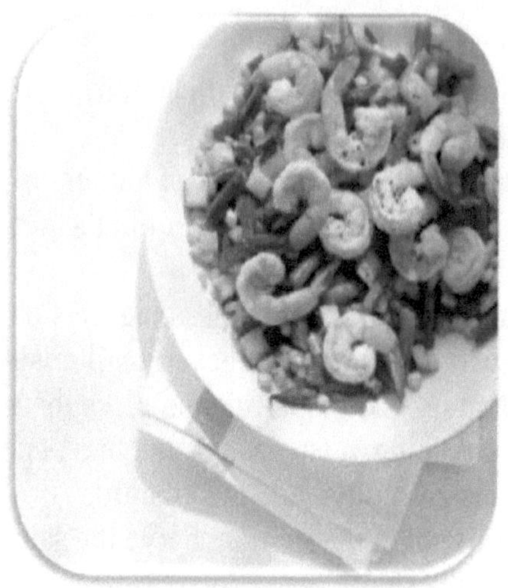

Prep time: 10 minutes
Cooking time: 25 minutes
Servings: 4

Nutrients per serving:

Carbohydrates – 26.8 g
Fat – 4.5 g
Protein – 37.3 g
Calories – 286

Ingredients:

- 2 slices natural, uncured bacon
- 1½ lbs peeled and deveined large shrimp
- ¾ tsp salt
- ½ tsp freshly ground black pepper
- 2 garlic cloves, minced
- 2 cups frozen lima beans, thawed
- 1 cup fresh corn kernels (about 2 ears)
- 1 (14.5-oz) can reduced-sodium chicken broth
- 2 cups chopped tomatoes
- ¼ cup fresh basil leaves

Instructions:

1. In a Dutch oven, cook the bacon for about 10 minutes. Remove the bacon, crumble it.
2. Sprinkle the shrimp with ½ tsp each of salt and pepper. Add the shrimp to the bacon drippings in the skillet, and cook, stirring occasionally, for 4 to 5 minutes. Keep warm.
3. Add the garlic to pan. Cook for 1 minute or until tender.
4. Add the lima beans, corn, chicken broth, and remaining ¼ tsp of salt.
5. Bring to a simmer.
6. Simmer, for 10 minutes or until the vegetables are tender.
7. Stir in the tomatoes, bacon, and basil. Cook for 1 minute. Serve hot.

Mighty Mushroom and Tilapia Seafood Dinner

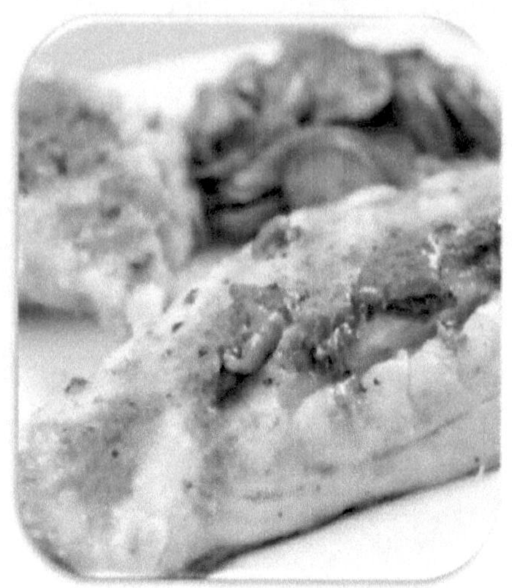

Prep time: 10 minutes
Cooking time: 15 minutes
Servings: 4

Nutrients per serving:

Carbohydrates – 2 g
Fat – 12 g
Protein – 43 g
Calories – 300

Ingredients:

- 4 medium-sized tilapia filets
- 2 Tbsp olive oil
- Juice from 1½ limes
- ½ tsp black pepper
- ½ tsp salt
- 3 minced garlic cloves
- 1 Tbsp sesame oil
- 1 Tbsp soy sauce
- 4 cups sliced button mushrooms

Instructions:

1. Preheat the broiler.
2. Place each of the tilapia filets on a baking sheet. Drizzle them with the olive oil and lime juice. Salt and pepper them as well.
3. Broil fillets for 4 minutes on each side.
4. In a skillet, add the sesame oil, garlic cloves and the mushrooms. Cook them for 5 minutes.
5. Add the soy sauce, and cook until all of the liquid is gone.
6. Serve the fish with the mushrooms on top.

Honey-Tamari Salmon with Rice and Snow Peas

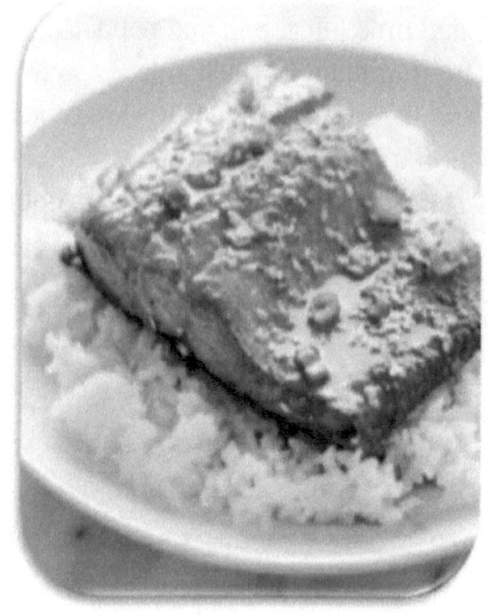

Prep time: 10 minutes
Cooking time: 15 minutes
Servings: 4

Nutrients per serving:

Carbohydrates – 59.1 g
Fat – 15.7 g
Protein – 46.2 g
Calories – 576

Ingredients:

- 3 Tbsp tamari or coconut aminos
- 2 Tbsp honey
- 1½ Tbsp brown rice vinegar
- 1 garlic clove, minced
- 1 tsp grated fresh ginger
- 1½ lbs center-cut salmon fillets
- 1 cup uncooked brown rice
- 1½ lbs snow peas, trimmed

Instructions:

1. In a bowl, whisk together the tamari, honey, vinegar, garlic, and ginger.
2. Place the salmon in a large zip-top plastic freezer bag.
3. Pour 3 Tbsp of the marinade over the salmon, reserve the rest. Marinate in the refrigerator for 15 minutes.
4. Cook the rice, then keep the rice warm.
5. Preheat the broiler.
6. Line a rimmed baking sheet with aluminum foil.
7. Place the salmon on the pan. Broil 5 inches from the heat for 8 to 10 minutes or until done.
8. Place the snow peas in a steamer basket in a pot with simmering water. Cover and steam for 3 minutes or until crisp-tender.
9. Place the salmon and rice on serving plates and drizzle with the reserved marinade. Serve with the snow peas.

Steamed Mussels in Tomato-Fennel Broth

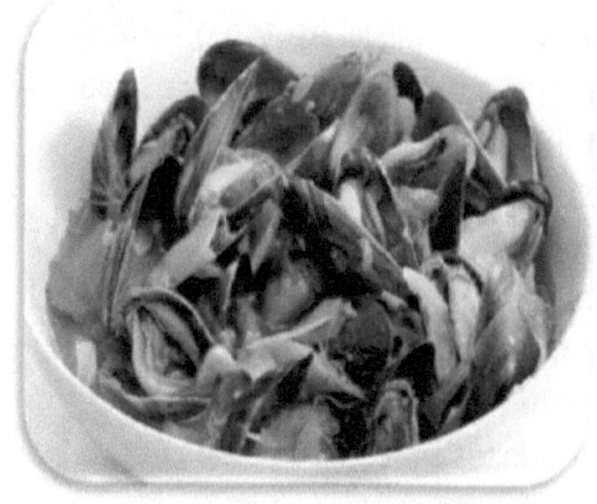

Prep time: 10 minutes
Cooking time: 30 minutes
Servings: 4

Nutrients per serving:

Carbohydrates – 51.6 g
Fat – 8.8 g
Protein – 35.4 g
Calories – 417

Ingredients:

- 2 Tbsp avocado oil
- 3 garlic cloves, minced
- 1 fennel bulb, thinly sliced, plus 2 Tbsp of the fennel fronds, chopped
- ½ cup fish stock
- 1 (28-oz) can whole tomatoes, chopped
- 2 Tbsp chopped fresh parsley
- ½ cup water
- 2 lbs mussels, scrubbed
- 8 oz 100% whole-grain French bread

Instructions:

1. In a Dutch oven, add the oil.
2. Add the garlic and fennel bulb slices. Cook for 8 minutes.

3. Add the fennel fronds and fish stock. Cook 2 minutes.
4. Add the tomatoes. Reduce the heat to low. Cover and simmer for 15 minutes.
5. Add the parsley, water, and mussels. Increase the temperature to medium-high. Cover and cook for 5 minutes.
6. Put the mussels in a large shallow bowl with the cooking liquid, discarding any unopened mussels.
7. Serve with thick slices of the French bread for dipping in the cooking liquid.

Chicken Pasta Puttanesca

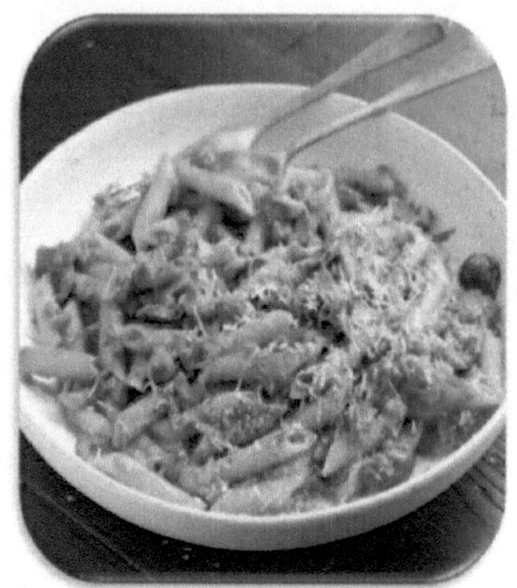

Prep time: 10 minutes
Cooking time: 20 minutes
Servings: 4

Nutrients per serving:

Carbohydrates – 76.1 g
Fat – 17.6 g
Protein – 63.6 g
Calories – 710

Ingredients:

- 12 oz 100% whole-grain penne
- 4 boneless skinless chicken breasts, cut into 1-inch pieces
- ½ tsp salt
- ½ tsp freshly ground black pepper
- 2 Tbsp avocado oil
- 2 garlic cloves, minced
- ¼ tsp crushed red pepper
- 1 (28-oz) can crushed tomatoes in puree
- ½ cup chopped pitted Kalamata olives
- 2 Tbsp capers

Instructions:

1. Cook the pasta, drain, and keep warm.
2. Sprinkle the chicken with salt and pepper.
3. Heat the oil in a Dutch oven.
4. Brown the chicken for 5 minutes, stirring occasionally
5. Add the garlic and crushed red pepper. Cook for 2 minutes.
6. Add the tomatoes, olives, and capers. Bring to a simmer. Cook for 5 minutes.
7. Add the pasta to the sauce; toss well to coat. Divide the chicken pasta among serving plates.

Tandoori Chicken Kabobs

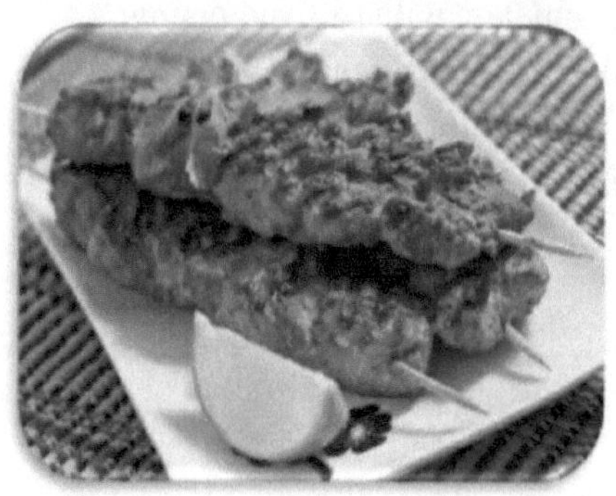

Prep time: 10 minutes
Cooking time: 10 minutes
Servings: 4

Nutrients per serving:

Carbohydrates – 5.7 g
Fat – 16.7 g
Protein – 56.8 g
Calories – 413

Ingredients:

- 1½ cups plain Greek yogurt
- 2 Tbsp lemon juice
- 2 tsp smoked paprika
- ½ tsp ground cumin
- ½ tsp ground coriander
- ½ tsp salt
- ½ tsp freshly ground black pepper
- ¼ tsp ground ginger
- ¼ tsp cayenne pepper
- 3 garlic cloves, minced
- 1½ lbs boneless skinless chicken breasts, cut into 2-inch cubes

Instructions:

1. In a medium bowl, whisk together the yogurt, lemon juice, paprika, cumin, coriander, salt, black pepper, ginger, cayenne pepper, and

garlic.
2. Place the chicken in a large zip-top plastic freezer bag. Add the yogurt mixture, turning to coat evenly.
3. Refrigerate covered for 4 to 8 hours.
4. Remove the chicken from the marinade.
5. Preheat the grill to medium-high heat.
6. Thread the chicken onto 8 12-inch skewers.
7. Grill the chicken for about 8 minutes, turning occasionally, or until done.
8. Serve the kabobs on the skewers

Pork and Bok Choy Stir-Fry

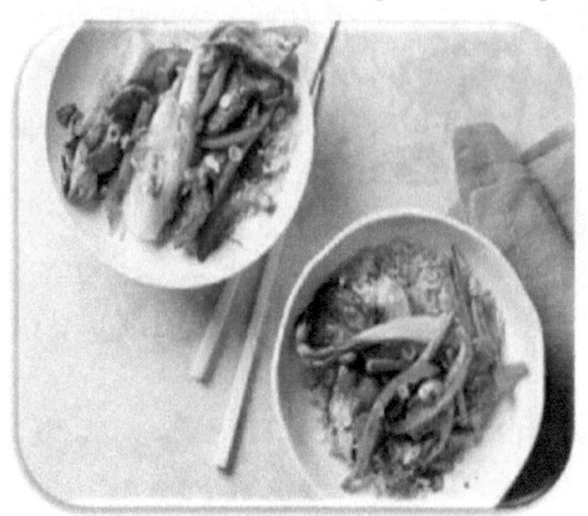

Prep time: 15 minutes
Cooking time: 40 minutes
Servings: 4

Nutrients per serving:

Carbohydrates – 66.7 g
Fat – 16 g
Protein – 45.3 g
Calories – 577

Ingredients:

- 1 cup uncooked brown rice
- 1 Tbsp arrowroot powder
- 1 Tbsp honey
- ¼ cup orange juice
- ¼ cup tamari
- 1 Tbsp brown rice vinegar
- 1 Tbsp dark sesame oil
- 1 Tbsp grated fresh ginger
- 2 garlic cloves, minced
- 2 Tbsp coconut oil
- 1 lb pork tenderloin, cut into thin strips
- 3 baby bok choy, cut into 1-inch pieces
- 1 red bell pepper, sliced

Instructions:

1. Cook the rice; keep warm.
2. In a small saucepan, whisk together the arrowroot powder, honey, orange juice, tamari, vinegar, sesame oil, ginger, and garlic. Cook on medium for 2 minutes. Set aside.
3. In a skillet over medium heat, heat 1 Tbsp of oil.
4. Add the pork to the skillet. Cook for 5 to 6 minutes.
5. Remove the pork from skillet and keep warm.
6. Heat the remaining 1 Tbsp of oil in the skillet.
7. Add the bok choy and bell pepper. Cook for 3 minutes or until crisp-tender.
8. Return pork and sauce to skillet, tossing to coat. Stir-fry completely.
9. Serve the pork and vegetables over the cooked rice.

Chicken and Broccoli Tetrazzini

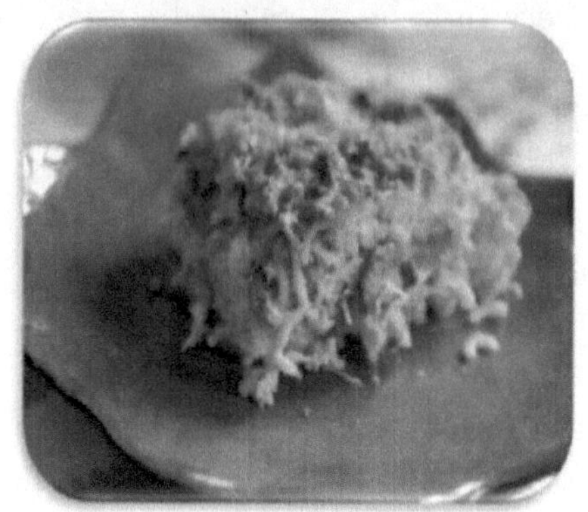

Prep time: 20 minutes
Cooking time: 40 minutes
Servings: 6

Nutrients per serving:

Carbohydrates – 28.4 g
Fat – 16 g
Protein – 31.2 g
Calories – 377

Ingredients:

- 3 Tbsp avocado oil, plus additional for greasing
- 1 (12-oz) package 100% whole-wheat spaghetti
- 1 (8-oz) package sliced fresh mushrooms
- ¼ cup 100% whole-wheat pastry flour
- 1 (14.5-oz) can reduced-sodium chicken broth
- 1 cup milk
- 1 cup freshly grated Parmesan cheese
- ½ tsp salt
- ½ tsp freshly ground black pepper
- 1 (16-oz) package frozen broccoli florets, thawed
- 2 cups shredded cooked chicken
- 1 cup sliced almonds

Instructions:

1. Preheat the oven to 400°F.
2. Coat a 13 x 9-inch baking dish with avocado oil.
3. Cook the pasta, drain, and keep warm.
4. Heat 1 Tbsp of oil in a nonstick skillet.
5. Add the mushrooms and cook 8 minutes or until browned and tender.
6. Heat the remaining 2 Tbsp of oil in the skillet.
7. Whisk in the flour. Cook for 1 minute or until bubbling.
8. Add the chicken broth. Bring to a boil and cook for 5 minutes.
9. Stir in the milk, ½ cup of cheese, salt, and pepper. Cook for 1 more minute.
10. In a bowl, combine the pasta, mushrooms, cream sauce, broccoli, and chicken.
11. Pour the mixture into prepared baking dish. Top with ½ cup of cheese and almonds.
12. Bake for 25 to 30 minutes, until casserole is browned and bubbly.
13. Cut the tetrazzini into squares and serve.

DESERTS

Banana Cookie with Choko Chips

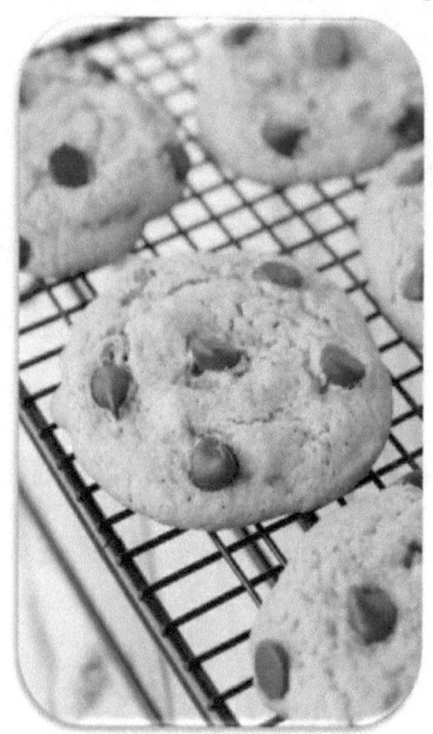

Prep time: 20 minutes
Cooking time: 25 minutes
Servings: 16

Nutrients per serving:

Carbohydrates – 20 g
Fat – 11 g
Protein – 2 g
Calories – 175

Ingredients:

- 4 mashed bananas
- 2 cups vegan chocolate chips
- 4 cups shredded unsweetened coconut

Instructions:

1. Preheat your oven to 350° F.
2. Combine the mashed bananas and the coconut.
3. Add the chocolate chips and stir well.
4. Form 32 cookies and drop them onto a cookie sheet.
5. Bake for 25 minutes.

Lemon-Lime Granita

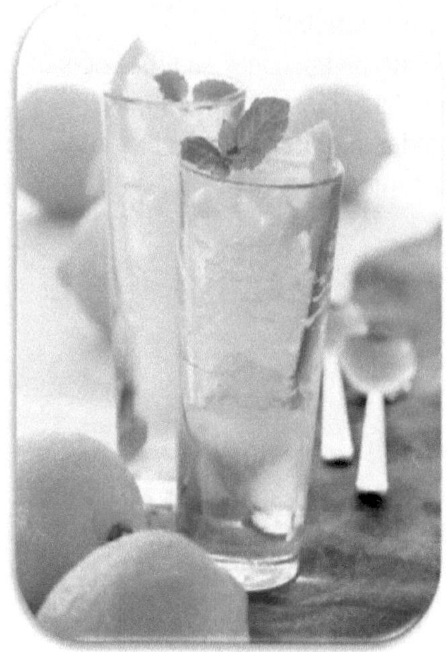

Prep time: 1 hour
Cooking time: none
Servings: 4

Nutrients per serving:

Carbohydrates – 19.1 g
Fat – 0.1 g
Protein – 0.3 g
Calories – 72

Ingredients:

- ¼ cup fresh lemon juice
- ¼ cup fresh lime juice
- 1 cup water
- ¼ cup liquid stevia
- 1 tsp fresh lemon zest
- 1 tsp fresh lemon rind

Instructions:

1. Combine all ingredients in a shallow metal baking dish.
2. Stir well, then place the dish in the freezer.
3. Stir the mixture with a fork every 10 to 15 minutes until it becomes slushy, about 45 minutes.
4. Once the granita is slushy, leave it in the freezer and scrape it around every 10 minutes until it has a crystallized, icy texture.
5. Spoon the granita into dessert cups and serve immediately.

Broiled Grapefruit with Honeyed Yogurt

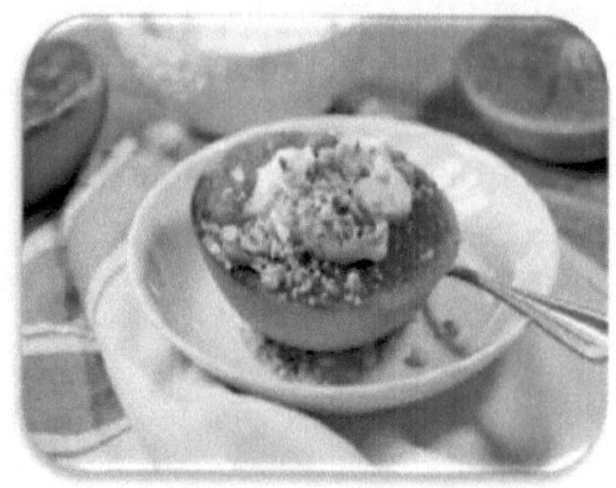

Prep time: 5 minutes
Cooking time: 10 minutes
Servings: 6

Nutrients per serving:

Carbohydrates – 26.7 g
Fat – 0.9 g
Protein – 2 g
Calories – 115

Ingredients:

- 3 ruby red grapefruits, halved and cut along the segments
- 6 Tbsp coconut sugar
- ¼ tsp ground cinnamon
- ½ cup plain Greek yogurt
- 3 Tbsp honey

Instructions:

1. Preheat the broiler to high.
2. Place the grapefruit halves, cut-side up, in a 13 x 9-inch baking pan.
3. Sprinkle the grapefruit with coconut sugar and cinnamon.
4. Broil for 5 minutes. Watch carefully so they don't burn. Remove to a wire rack to cool a bit.
5. In a small bowl, stir together the yogurt and honey. Dollop it evenly on warm grapefruit halves.
6. Serve warm.

Apple Crumble

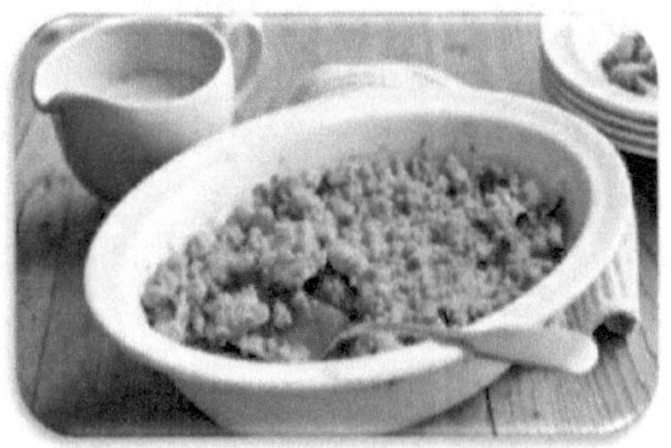

Prep time: 10 minutes
Cooking time: 20 minutes
Servings: 6

Nutrients per serving:

Carbohydrates – 26.9 g
Fat – 6.5 g
Protein – 2.5 g
Calories – 167

Ingredients:

- Coconut oil, for greasing
- 4 apples, peeled and thinly sliced
- 3 Tbsp lemon juice
- ½ tsp pure vanilla extract
- 4 Tbsp evaporated cane juice, divided
- 1 tsp ground cinnamon
- ¼ tsp ground nutmeg
- 7 Tbsp 100% whole-wheat pastry flour, divided
- ½ cup uncooked old-fashioned rolled oats
- ¼ cup chopped almonds
- 2 Tbsp cold butter, cut into pieces

Instructions:

1. Preheat the oven to 375°F.
2. Coat an 8-inch square baking pan with coconut oil.
3. In a medium bowl, toss together the apples, lemon juice, vanilla, 1 Tbsp of evaporated cane juice, ½ tsp of cinnamon, nutmeg, and 1

Tbsp of flour.

4. Pour the mixture into the prepared baking pan.
5. In another bowl, stir together the remaining 6 Tbsp of flour, oats, the remaining cinnamon, the remaining cane juice, almonds, and butter. Mix until crumbly.
6. Spoon the crumble mixture over the apples.
7. Bake for 25 minutes. Serve warm.

Apple-Raisin Rice Pudding

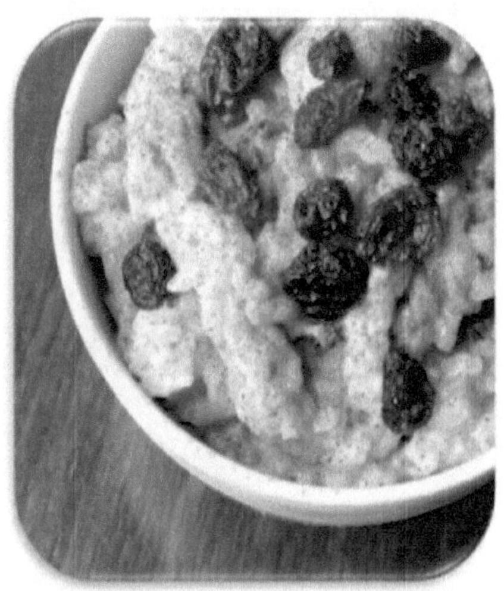

Prep time: 30 minutes
Cooking time: 40 minutes
Servings: 4

Nutrients per serving:

Carbohydrates – 49 g
Fat – 4.5 g
Protein – 8.1 g
Calories – 264

Ingredients:

- 3 cups milk
- ½ cup short-grain brown rice
- ¼ cup pure maple syrup
- ¼ cup raisins
- ¼ cup dried apples
- Pinch salt
- 1 tsp pure vanilla extract
- 1 tsp ground cinnamon

Instructions:

1. In a saucepan, combine the milk, rice, maple syrup, raisins, apples,

and salt.
2. Bring to a boil, stirring frequently to prevent scorching.
3. Reduce the heat to low and simmer for 20 minutes, stirring frequently.
4. Stir in the vanilla and cinnamon.
5. Serve warm.

Yogurt Cheesecake Bars with Berry Topping

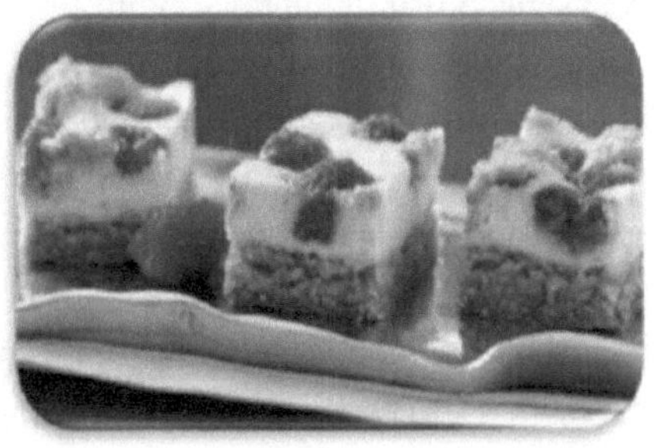

Prep time: 20 minutes
Cooking time: 40 minutes
Servings: 8

Nutrients per serving:

Carbohydrates – 36.6 g
Fat – 22.9 g
Protein – 7.3 g
Calories – 379

Ingredients:

- Coconut oil, for greasing
- ¾ cup uncooked old-fashioned rolled oats
- ¼ cup almond flour
- 1 tsp ground cinnamon
- 4½ Tbsp coconut sugar, divided
- 1½ Tbsp butter, melted
- 1½ Tbsp unsweetened almond milk
- 1 (8-oz) package cream cheese, softened
- ¼ cup honey
- 2 eggs
- 1 Tbsp pure vanilla extract
- 1 tsp lemon zest
- 1 cup plain Greek yogurt
- 1 cup warm berry sauce

Instructions:

1. Preheat the oven to 325°F.

2. Coat an 8-inch square pan with coconut oil.
3. In a food processor, pulse the oats, almond flour, cinnamon, and 2½ Tbsp of coconut sugar until coarsely ground.
4. Add the butter and milk; pulse until the mixture resembles wet crumbs.
5. Press the crust into the prepared pan.
6. Bake for 8 minutes or until set. Let cool slightly.
7. In a bowl, beat the cream cheese, honey, and remaining 2 Tbsp coconut sugar with a mixer at medium speed until fluffy.
8. Add the eggs, beating until the yellow disappears.
9. Add the vanilla, lemon zest, and yogurt and beat just until combined.
10.   Pour the filling over the prepared crust. Bake for 35 minutes.
11.   Remove the cheesecake from the oven and cool completely.
12.   Refrigerate the cheesecake for 3 hours or until chilled; cut into squares. Serve with the sauce spooned over the squares.

Quick Vanilla Pudding

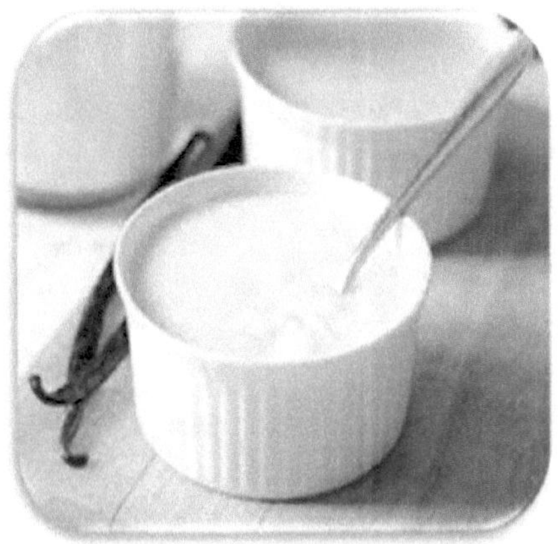

Prep time: 5 minutes
Cooking time: 5 minutes
Servings: 4

Nutrients per serving:

Carbohydrates – 15.7 g
Fat – 3.8 g
Protein – 5 g
Calories – 122

Ingredients:

- 2 Tbsp arrowroot powder
- 2 cups milk
- 2 Tbsp evaporated cane juice
- 1 Tbsp pure vanilla extract
- 1 egg yolk

Instructions:

1. In a saucepan, whisk together the arrowroot and milk until no lumps remain.
2. Whisk in the cane juice and vanilla extract.
3. Bring the mixture to a simmer. Cook for 1 to 2 minutes.
4. Place the egg yolk in a small bowl. Add 1 Tbsp of the hot milk mixture, whisking constantly so the egg yolk doesn't cook.

5. Add another 1 Tbsp of hot milk mixture and whisk again.
6. Then, whisking constantly, pour the milk-egg yolk mixture into the thickened hot milk. Cook for 1 minute.
7. Divide the pudding among dessert dishes and refrigerate until set, at least 1 hour.
8. Serve chilled.

Dark Cherry, Pistachio, Coconut, and Bittersweet Chocolate Bark

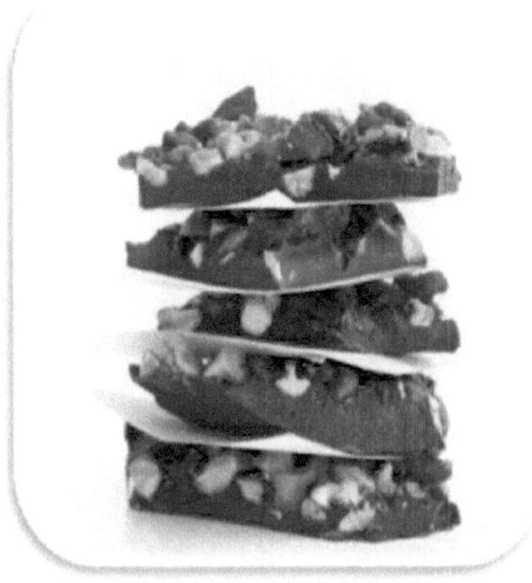

Prep time: 5 minutes
Cooking time: 5 minutes
Servings: 16

Nutrients per serving:

Carbohydrates – 21.6 g
Fat – 10.3 g
Protein – 3.8 g
Calories – 185

Ingredients:

- 12 oz 70% bittersweet chocolate, chopped
- 1 cup coarsely chopped unsalted pistachios, shelled
- 1 cup dried unsweetened cherries
- ¼ cup toasted shredded unsweetened coconut
- ½ tsp coarse sea salt

Instructions:

1. Line a baking sheet with parchment paper.
2. In a bowl over a saucepan of simmering water, melt the chocolate, stirring frequently, until smooth and melted, about 5 minutes.
3. Pour the chocolate onto the baking sheet, spreading it to about ¼

inch thickness.

4. Top evenly with the pistachios, cherries, coconut, and salt.
5. Chill until the bark is firm, about 30 minutes.
6. Remove the parchment paper and break the chocolate into pieces.
7. Store the bark in the refrigerator in an airtight container for up to 1 month.

Dark Chocolate Bread Puddings

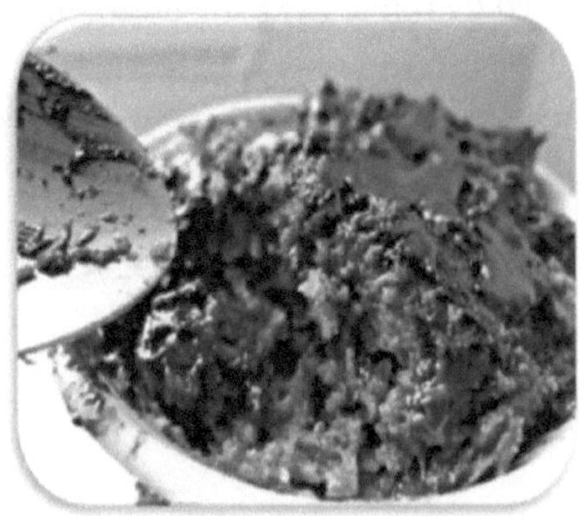

Prep time: 15 minutes
Cooking time: 25 minutes
Servings: 12

Nutrients per serving:

Carbohydrates – 27 g
Fat – 5.2 g
Protein – 8.7 g
Calories – 227

Ingredients:

- Coconut oil, for greasing
- 3 cups milk
- 4 eggs, lightly beaten
- ¾ cup evaporated cane juice
- 2 Tbsp unsweetened cocoa powder
- ½ tsp pure vanilla extract
- 12 oz 100% whole-grain bread, cut into 1-inch pieces
- 8 oz 70% bittersweet chocolate, chopped

Instructions:

1. Preheat the oven to 350°F.
2. Coat 12 cups of a standard muffin tin with coconut oil.
3. In a bowl, whisk together the milk, eggs, cane juice, cocoa powder, and vanilla.

4. Add the bread and chocolate. Let stand for 10 minutes.
5. Fill the prepared muffin tin with the bread mixture. Bake for 25 minutes, or until set.
6. Serve warm, or cool and refrigerate, covered, for 3 days.

Fudgy Chocolate Chunk-Pecan Brownies

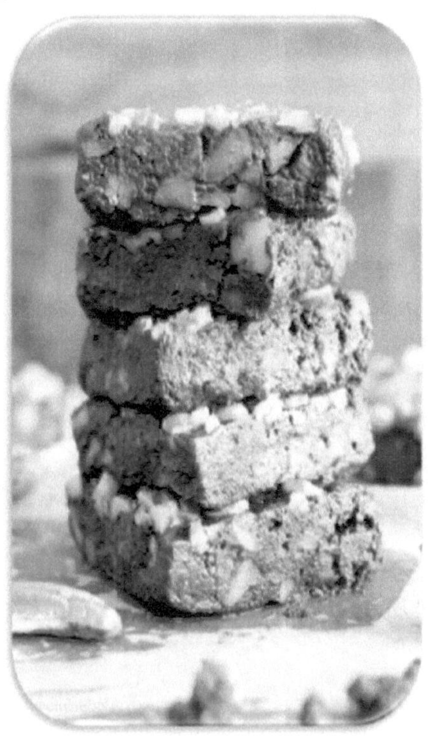

Prep time: 15 minutes
Cooking time: 25 minutes
Servings: 12

Nutrients per serving:

Carbohydrates – 23.5 g
Fat – 11.7 g
Protein – 2.5 g
Calories – 199

Ingredients:

- Coconut oil, for greasing
- ½ cup butter, melted
- 1 cup coconut sugar
- 1 tsp pure vanilla extract
- 2 eggs
- 1 cup unsweetened cocoa powder

- ½ cup 100% whole-wheat pastry flour
- ¼ tsp baking powder
- ¼ tsp salt
- ½ cup chopped 70% bittersweet chocolate
- ½ cup toasted chopped pecans

Instructions:

1. Preheat the oven to 350°F.
2. Coat a 9-inch square baking pan with coconut oil.
3. In a medium bowl, stir together the butter, sugar, vanilla extract, and eggs.
4. In another bowl, whisk together the cocoa powder, pastry flour, baking powder, salt, chocolate, and pecans.
5. Add the dry mixture to the butter mixture, stirring just until combined.
6. Spread the batter into the prepared pan. Bake for about 20 minutes. Serve warm or at room temperature.

Conversion Tables

VOLUME EQUIVALENTS (LIQUID)

US STANDARD	US STANDARD (OUNCES)	METRIC
2 tablespoons	1 fl. oz.	30 mL
¼ cup	2 fl. oz.	60 mL
½ cup	4 fl. oz.	120 mL
1 cup	8 fl. oz.	240mL
1½ cups	12 fl. oz.	355 mL
2 cups or 1 pint	16 fl. oz.	475 mL
4 cups or 1 quart	32 fl. oz.	1 L
1 gallon	128 fl. oz.	4 L

OVEN TEMPERATURES

FAHRENHEIT (°F)	CELSIUS (°C) APPROXIMATE
250 °F	120 °C
300 °F	150 °C
325 °F	165 °C
350 °F	180 °C
375 °F	190 °C
400 °F	200 °C
425 °F	220 °C
450 °F	230 °C

VOLUME EQUIVALENTS (LIQUID)

US STANDARD	METRIC (APPROXIMATE)
1/8 teaspoon	0.5 mL
¼ teaspoon	1 mL
½ teaspoon	2 mL
2/3 teaspoon	4 mL
1 teaspoon	5 mL
1 tablespoon	15 mL
¼ cup	59 mL
1/3 cup	79 mL
½ cup	118 mL
2/3 cup	156 mL
¾ cup	177 mL
1 cup	235 mL
2 cups or 1 pint	475 mL
3 cups	700 mL
4 cups or 1 quart	1 L
½ gallon	2 L
1 gallon	4 L

WEIGHT EQUIVALENTS

US STANDARD	METRIC (APPROXIMATE)
½ ounce	15 g
1 ounce	30 g
2 ounces	60 g
4 ounces	115 g
8 ounces	225 g
12 ounces	340 g
16 ounces or 1 pound	455 g